Exercise for Older Adults

ACE'S GUIDE FOR FITNESS PROFESSIONALS

TABLE OF
contents

reviewers

Susan J. Bartlett, Ph.D., is a post-doctoral fellow at Johns Hopkins School of Medicine, and a clinical psychologist at the Johns Hopkins Weight Management Center in Baltimore, Md. Dr. Bartlett authored two chapters of the ACE Lifestyle & Weight Management Consultant Manual.

Jennifer S. Bolger, M.S., received her masters in exercise physiology from San Diego State University. She is the Fitness Program Director at the Mission Valley YMCA in San Diego, Calif. It is there that she developed the 12-week Personalized Fitness Program, which is designed to help underactive adults make a behavior change to include regular physical activity into their lives.

John L. Boyer, M.D., is a past president of the American College of Sports Medicine and an Emeritus Professor in the College of Professional Studies at San Diego State University. He has a 35-year background in medicine and cardiology with emphasis on risk-factor modification in the prevention and rehabilitation of cardiovascular disorders.

Lawrence J. Cheskin, M.D., F.A.C.P., is an associate professor of medicine and director of the Johns Hopkins Weight Management Center. He is the author of Losing Weight for Good: Develop Your Personal Plan of Action (Johns Hopkins Press), as well as a board-certified gastroenterologist.

Laura A. Gladwin, M.S., is the president of LGA Fitness Consulting & Training, Brea, Calif., a firm that provides training in the development of senior fitness/wellness programming to fitness professionals and organizations worldwide. She also serves on the National Coalition for Developing Curriculum Standards for Senior Fitness Specialists (SFA), the advisory board for SFA, is director of Senior Fitness for AFAA, and is a member of the advisory board and teaching staff for the Senior Fitness Certificate Program at California State University, Fullerton.

Jeanne F. Nichols, Ph.D., is a professor of exercise physiology in the Department of Exercise and Nutritional Sciences and director of the Adult Fitness Program at San Diego State University.

Brenda L. Wolfe, Ph.D., is a psychologist who specializes in designing self-help programs. She is currently president of Self Management Systems, Inc., affiliated with the University of New Mexico, and travels nationally training health professionals in lifestyle intervention techniques. She also has served as director of research for Jenny Craig Weight Loss Centres, published in both the popular and professional press, and is a recent past-chair of the Obesity and Eating Disorders Special Interest Group of the Association for Advancement of Behavior Therapy.

foreword

Until recently, a large segment of our society was left out of the fitness revolution that began in the '70s, gained steam in the '80s and hit its stride in the '90s. This revolution was aimed primarily at the young and fit. But that neglected segment of society—older adults—has since increased in both strength and number. While fewer than 4 percent of adults were older than 65 at the turn of the century, the number of people older than 65 in the year 2020 will reach an estimated 51 million.

Modern medicine, a better understanding of disease and improved nutrition are largely responsible for this expected demographic shift. But these numbers say nothing about the quality of life those who live past 65 can expect. This is where the role of lifestyle and physical activity come into play. Numerous studies have demonstrated the power of physical activity to not only extend one's life, but to enhance the ability to carry on with activities of daily living. These are the things we all take for granted in our youth—caring for ourselves and others, living independently, even dressing and feeding ourselves—that can drastically alter one's ability to enjoy life should disease or disability take over.

Young or old, there is no question that physical activity can significantly improve the quality of one's life. But the type and intensity of that activity may change depending on one's age. To better answer the unique needs of older adults, the American Council on Exercise created the book you now hold in your hands: *Exercise for Older Adults: ACE's Guide for Fitness Professionals.* It offers the essential information fitness professionals need to provide older adults with safe and effective fitness programming, from the physiology of aging to the techniques and tools for motivating and communicating with older adults.

Working with older adults is rich with opportunities for both personal and professional rewards. In many cases, this is an untapped market with many communities, groups and individuals previously overlooked by the fitness industry. But on a personal level, the benefits run even deeper. Introducing physical activity to an older adult may literally make the difference between life and death or, at the very least, make a major difference in the quality of that individual's life. Take advantage of the opportunity this manual affords you—expand your scope of knowledge, hone your skills and increase your understanding to better serve the older adult community.

Sheryl Marks Brown
Executive Director

introduction

Exercise for Older Adults: ACE's Guide for Fitness Professionals presents the most current, complete picture of the knowledge, instructional and communication techniques that fitness professionals who work with older adults need to provide safe and effective exercise programming for their clients. It is designed to serve as a comprehensive resource to help you in your day-to-day practice.

We brought together top experts from the fields of exercise physiology and psychology who specialize in the specific needs of older adults to develop a manual that meets the growing demand for clear and comprehensive guidelines for fitness professionals who wish to better serve this growing community. Each chapter is a building block of knowledge, arranged logically to give you an understanding of the basic principles and skills inherent to working with older adults.

The physiological and functional changes associated with aging and their effects on exercise are detailed in Chapter 1, while Chapter 2 explores the most effective ways to communicate with older adults. Specific, insightful methods to encourage the adoption of healthful habits are given, as well as insight on how to help clients set goals and provide sufficient motivation to achieve them.

Building upon the knowledge gained in Chapter 1, Chapter 3 covers age-related medical conditions and, most importantly, how to adapt exercise programs accordingly. The physiological and psychological effects of medications common to older adults also are discussed. Chapter 4 offers a comprehensive assessment protocol, with a broad range of tools to improve information gathering.

Even very fit older adults are likely to have different tastes and requirements regarding the types of activities they find enjoyable. Chapter 5 presents a variety of modes and techniques appropriate for an older population. From warm-up to cool-down, this chapter includes comprehensive guidelines and ideas for modifications, and includes options for both chair-based and water-based exercises.

Finally, Chapter 6 explains how to use the pre-exercise assessment results to structure both individual and group exercise programs for seniors, as well as how to lead older clients and class members in cardiovascular, strength and flexibility training.

Whether you are an activity director, personal trainer, health educator or fitness facility manager, you will benefit from this valuable resource. If you are familiar with the older adult population, you understand the challenge and rewards that come from focusing on this under-served group. Your challenge is to learn how to apply this information in a way that is appealing, brings about results, and ensures the long-term success of your older adult clients. In addition to enriching and expanding your career, your rewards come from not only helping older adults achieve their personal fitness goals, but live healthier lives as well.

Richard T. Cotton
Editor

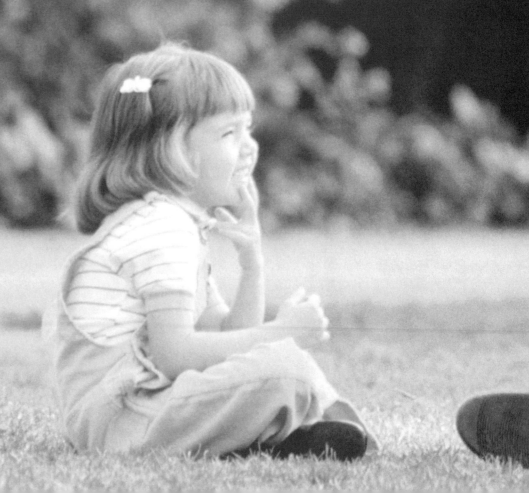

PHYSIOLOGY OF
aging and exercise

Wojtek J. Chodzko-Zajko

Wojtek J. Chodzko-Zajko, Ph.D., B.Ed. is an associate professor in the School of Exercise, Leisure and Sport at Kent State University where he has established an ongoing longitudinal study of exercise and aging. Chodzko-Zajko serves on the Scientific Advisory Committee of the World Health Organization, which recently issued Guidelines for Physical Activity in Older Adults, and has published in the areas of physiology of aging, cognitive changes in aging, and age changes in sensory and motor functioning. Dr. Chodzko-Zajko also is editor of the Journal of Aging and Physical Activity.

Aging is a universal phenomenon that affects us all. Provided we live long enough, we will eventually experience significant sensory, motor and cognitive changes in response to advancing age. However, although we are all aging, we do not age at the same rate. While some people experience relatively rapid declines in physiological and psychological functioning as they grow older, others undergo significantly less-pronounced changes over time (Fries & Crapo, 1981).

In recent years, **gerontologists** have focused on increasing our understanding of the factors responsible for individual differences in the rate and extent at which we age. Clearly, hereditary factors play an important role in determining the pattern of changes observed in **senescence.** This genetic component of human aging is largely beyond our control and gerontologists often joke that the single best way to ensure longevity and healthful old age is to choose one's parents wisely! However, in addition to the genetic factors influencing human aging, there is now strong evidence that many aspects of the aging process are related to environmental factors, such as nutrition, stress, smoking and physical activity (Bokovy & Blair, 1994).

The need to develop effective lifestyle interventions that have the potential to improve the quality of life for older persons is especially apparent when one considers the growing proportion of older adults in today's society. Whereas individuals older than 65 constituted a mere four percent of the American population in 1900, they now represent more than 12 percent of the population (Gerber, 1989). Available evidence strongly suggests that this growth rate will continue. The Census Bureau predicts that by the year 2010 there will be approximately 39 million people older than 65. By 2020, the number of those 65 and older will rise to 51 million—nearly 20 percent of the population (U.S. Census Bureau, 1990). Even more remarkable is the increase in the number of the oldest members of our society—termed the "old-old." By the year 2030, it is anticipated that more than 8 million Americans will be 85 or older (Fowles, 1991).

There is little doubt that such a dramatic increase in the number of older adults will have far-reaching consequences for society. The past two decades have witnessed a remarkable expansion of interest in the physical activity needs of older persons. The major medical and scientific organizations endorse the importance of physically active lifestyles for older adults (ACSM, 1995; U.S. Surgeon General, 1996; World Health Organization, 1997). It is now possible for students to specialize in the study of physical activity and aging, both through traditional academic programs offered at universities (Jones & Rikli, 1994), and special-

ized programs such as those offered by the American Council on Exercise.

This chapter examines some of the key issues influencing the relationship between physical activity and the aging process. We begin with a discussion of underlying biological mechanisms responsible for aging, including: 1) What is aging? 2) What causes us to age? 3) What are the consequences of aging? and 4) Why do some people appear to age faster than others? We then examine the role regular physical activity plays in physiological, psychological and social functioning, and the extent to which lifestyle change promotes healthy aging. Finally, we discuss issues related to the prescription of exercise for older persons. Throughout the chapter a broad definition of physical activity is adopted, and the *acute* or short-term effects of a single bout of activity and the *chronic* or long-term benefits of extended participation are considered.

The Physiology of the Aging Process

Aging Defined

It may seem unnecessary to define aging. Age is typically defined as the number of years, months or days that have elapsed since a particular point in time, usually birth. Similarly, the *aging process* is almost always defined by the passage of calendar time. However, many gerontologists believe definitions of aging that focus exclusively on calendar time are incomplete, and that more complex definitions of both "age" and "aging" are needed to understand the intricacies associated with human aging.

Chronological age is the length of time—expressed by the number of years or months since birth—a person has lived. Its measurement is independent of physiological, psychological and socio-cultural factors. The presence of large differences in functional performance between individuals of the same chronological age, however, suggests that chronological age alone is an insufficient measure of senescence.

Many gerontologists believe that to increase our understanding of senescence, chronological age must be supplemented by other measures of aging designed to differentiate between individuals of the same chronological age. These measures are often described as indices of **functional age.** The most common measure of functional age is biological age, although other functional ages, including psychological age and social age, have been identified (Schroots & Birren, 1990).

Biological age characterizes senescence in terms of discrete biological, rather than chronological, processes. Research designs that emphasize chronological age typically focus on elements of calendar time (years, decades, etc.) as the principal units of analysis, whereas biological-age research focuses on senescent changes in biological or physiological processes and their subsequent effects on behavior. A common goal of all biological age inventories is to determine **relative age,** or the extent to which an individual is aging faster or slower than an average person of the same chronological age. For example, an individual who is aging successfully may have a biological age 10 years younger than their chronological age. Conversely, a person experiencing multiple medical problems in old age may be biologically older than they are chronologically.

Because there is little consensus as to how biological age should be measured, it is difficult to summarize the research on the effects of physical activity on biological age. However, most studies suggest that, on average, people who exercise regularly have lower biological ages than people of the same chronological age who do not exercise (Chodzko-Zajko & Ringel, 1987; Heikkinen et al., 1994; Kim & Tanaka, 1995).

In much the same way that people of the same chronological age can differ biologically, it also is possible for people to have different psychological ages (Schroots & Birren, 1990). **Psychological age** refers to an individual's capabilities along a number of dimensions of mental or cognitive functioning, including self-esteem and self-efficacy, as well as learning, memory and perception (Birren, 1959). Birren suggests that some older persons demonstrate psychological adjustments typical for their chronological age, whereas others behave as though they were psychologically younger or older than their contemporaries. The concept of psychological age and its relationship to quality of life is now an important area of exercise science research. Recognizing the importance of regular physical activity in the psychological, social and physiological health of older persons, the World Health Organization (WHO) published the *Guidelines for Promoting Physical Activity Among Older Persons* in 1997.

Social age refers to the notion that society often has fairly rigid expectations of what is and is not appropriate behavior for a person of a particular age (Rose, 1972; McGrath & Kelly, 1985). Socialization is a tremendously complex process, and it is difficult to make broad generalizations about the acquisition of social roles in later life (McPherson, 1990). However, the impact that social roles and expectations have on the lifestyle choices of older persons is of considerable interest in experimental gerontology. A number of recent studies have examined the extent to which later-life physical activity choices are dependent on an individual's perception of what is, or is not, age-appropriate behavior (Cousins & Vertinsky, 1995; Cousins, 1997). For example, many older persons consider it undignified to be seen physically exerting themselves in public. The WHO guidelines encourage older people to break away from such stereotypical perspectives about aging. Instead of encouraging seniors to "take it easy," the WHO promotes a more vigorous and healthful model of aging in which older persons are invited to play a more active role in their own senescence (WHO, 1997).

Unfortunately, despite many years of research, there is no consensus on how best to quantify any of these alternative measures of aging. Thus, although it is apparent that chronological age is an inadequate measure of senescence and that alternative definitions of aging are necessary, no single unified definition of biological, psychological or social aging exists (Balin, 1994). Nonetheless, it is clear that an appreciation of chronological, biological and psychosocial perspectives on aging is essential to grasp the true essence of aging.

A central tenet underlying physical fitness and aging research is that physically fit individuals may be functionally younger than less-fit individuals of the same chronological age. From this point of view, research studies examining the relationship between age, physical fitness and behavior focus on both chronological and functional perspectives on aging.

Biological Theories of Aging

Biological theories of aging examine the underlying mechanisms responsible for the structural and functional changes that characterize advancing age. Researchers have attempted to specify a single causal element responsible for age-related declines in physiological functioning but, to date, little progress has been made toward identifying a unified theory of biological

aging (Hayflick, 1985; Baker & Martin, 1994).

Aging is probably not a single biological process, but rather a wide variety of age-related changes that occur simultaneously in many different systems throughout the body. Together, these changes decrease the body's ability to respond appropriately to the stresses of everyday life (Chodzko-Zajko & Ringel, 1987).

The complex nature of aging is reflected by the wide variety of theories proposed to account for the underlying mechanisms of aging. While many different classification schemes exist (Arking, 1991), the model proposed by the renowned biologist Leonard Hayflick is among the most straightforward (Hayflick, 1985). Hayflick was one of the first to demonstrate conclusively that cellular aging is influenced by both genetic and environmental factors. In his model of biological aging, Hayflick proposes that aging theories can be subdivided into three major classes: cellular theories, genetic theories and control theories.

Cellular Theories of Aging

Cellular theories of aging focus on the degenerative changes that occur at the level of the individual cell. The most commonly proposed mechanism of cellular aging is **free-radical oxidation** (Harman, 1956). A free radical is a highly unstable molecule of oxygen with an uneven number of electrons in its outer shell. The presence of an unpaired electron causes the oxygen-free radical to be both unstable and highly chemically reactive. To obtain the electron it needs to achieve stability, the free radical attempts to link up with other molecules. This process initiates a cascade of destructive chain reactions that may number in the thousands.

In healthy individuals, free radicals coexist in a state of equilibrium with a series of mixed-function oxidases that neutralize the destructive effects. The disruption of this equilibrium may be caused by a wide variety of intrinsic biological processes, as well as in response to environmental factors, such as exposure to radiation and chemical carcinogens. It is now well established that advancing age is associated with a reduction in the expression of mixed-function oxidases, which in turn leads to a progressive increase in free-radical oxidation (Balin, 1983; Baker & Martin, 1994). Alterations to the structure of collagen and elastin, the destruction of DNA, and a progressive breakdown of the immune system are among the damages attributed to free radicals (Arking, 1991).

The formation of covalent and hydrogen bond cross-links between adjacent molecules is a consequence of age-related increases in free-radical oxidation (Bjorksten, 1968). The bonding of adjacent molecules alters their configuration and has significant functional consequences. For example, age-related changes in skin elasticity may be the result of the formation of cross-links caused by increases in free-radical oxidation (Partridge, 1970). Aging also is associated with significant declines in flexibility and range of motion (Vandervoort et al., 1992), and it is likely that these changes are due, in part, to intrinsic changes brought about by cellular aging.

Genetic Theories of Aging

Genetic theories of aging focus on the role of heredity in the regulation of senescence. Studies of identical twins reveal that a significant portion of age-related changes in physiological variables can be attributed to genetic mechanisms (Kallman, 1948). Medvedev (1981) proposed that aging is the result of a breakdown in the integrity of DNA nucleotide sequences. This loss of DNA sequences disrupts the ability of the cell to reproduce. Although some degree of

DNA mutation occurs at all stages of the life cycle, the adverse consequences of these mutations are seldom realized until later in life.

Hayflick proposed that senescence is controlled by a purposeful sequence of events written into the genetic code (Hayflick, 1965; 1985). He showed that cells cultured in vitro exhibit a finite ability to reproduce. The **Hayflick limit** has been replicated in numerous tissues from a wide variety of species (Hayflick, 1985), and suggests that cellular aging is, at least to some extent, preprogrammed.

Hayflick's finding indicates that, although important, lifestyle changes alone will not allow us to overcome the genetically programmed factors responsible for human aging. We cannot escape the aging process indefinitely.

Control Theories of Aging

A third class of theories explains aging in terms of the function of specific systems known to be vital for the control of physiological functioning. For example, it is now accepted that advancing age often compromises immune system functioning. Older persons not only exhibit a significant decline in T-cell activity, but they also are more susceptible to autoimmune disease (Walford, 1987).

The **Major Histocompatibility Complex (MHC)** is a complex series of genes that provides a viable link between the cellular, genetic and control theories of aging. The MHC not only controls immunologic functioning, but also regulates the expression of mixed-function oxidases, which protect cells against damaging free-radical oxidation (Walford, 1983). Walford showed that genetic control of the immune system occurs in the MHC, the integrity of which typically deteriorates with advancing age (Walford, 1987). In addition to the immune system, the neuroendocrine and central nervous systems also have been implicated in the regulation of degenerative changes in aging (Arking, 1991; Baker & Martin, 1994). Future research will likely confirm the importance of several different control systems in the regulation of aging at the molecular, cellular and intact-organ levels.

Available evidence suggests that biological aging is a complex process regulated by numerous, redundant mechanisms. It is unlikely that a single biological mechanism can be identified as the principal factor responsible for senescence. Rather, it is more probable that a complex combination of mechanisms, acting at several different levels throughout the body, bring about the structural and functional changes that characterize old age. Since biological aging does not appear to be caused by a single mechanism, it is extremely unlikely that we will develop a "cure" for the aging process in the foreseeable future.

The Structural and Functional Consequences of Aging

The structural and functional consequences of aging are surprisingly consistent across a broad range of physiological systems. A General Model of Aging (Figure 1.1) summarizes the common structural and functional changes that are characteristic of aging throughout the body (Chodzko-Zajko & Ringel, 1987).

With advancing age, most physiological systems eventually exhibit atrophy, dystrophy and edema at the cellular level. These disruptions in the integrity of the cell are, in turn, precursors of more gross morphological changes, such as decreased elasticity and compliance, **demyelinization** and **neoplastic** growth. As expected, these structural changes are almost always associated with profound behavioral consequences.

In much the same way that structural changes exhibit similarities across physiological systems, the functional consequences also are fairly consistent across different systems of the body. Aging organ systems, which are usually slower and less accurate, exhibit not only reduced strength and stability, but also decreased coordination and endurance.

Although structural decay and functional decline are an inescapable consequence of aging, both the rate and extent of this decline vary widely between individuals. Individuals may deviate from expected patterns of aging and, at least for some period of time, postpone the consequences of aging (Fries & Crapo, 1981). For example, while measures of cardiovascular functioning usually decline with age

Figure 1.1

General Model of Aging

Structural Changes	Functional Consequences
Atrophy ($\uparrow$)	Accuracy ($\downarrow$)
Dystrophy ($\uparrow$)	Speed ($\downarrow$)
Edema ($\uparrow$)	Range ($\downarrow$)
Elasticity ($\downarrow$)	Endurance ($\downarrow$)
Demyelinization ($\uparrow$)	Coordination ($\downarrow$)
Neoplasm ($\uparrow$)	Stability ($\downarrow$)
Mutation ($\uparrow$)	Strength ($\downarrow$)

(Chodzko-Zajko & Ringel, 1987)

(Lakatta, 1990), physically fit and active individuals sometimes exhibit slower declines in function than less healthy people of the same age (Goldberg & Hagberg, 1990). Researchers at San Diego State University studied a group of regular exercisers for several decades. Declines in maximal oxygen consumption were considerably less than the 10-percent-per-decade decrease that is usually observed in the general population (Kasch et al., 1990).

The physiological consequences of aging cannot be offset indefinitely. Nonetheless, there is increasingly strong evidence to suggest that aging need not occur at a uniform rate. Indeed, many age-related changes may be modified by specific lifestyle interventions, including regular physical activity.

Lifestyle Interventions— Regular Physical Activity

The Benefits of Exercise for Older Adults

A good deal of attention has focused on the importance of regular physical activity as a means of enhancing health and effective functioning in old age. While most early research has focused on relatively young and healthy adults, there is now a conscious effort to extend our knowledge to a broader cross-section of the population. As understanding of the physiological, psychological and sociocultural significance of exercise grows, an increasing proportion of adults are opting to participate in some form of structured physical activity. Physicians and other health-care professionals are now recommending exercise as an adjunct to more traditional therapy for a variety of physical and psychological disorders.

Two recently published reports strongly endorse participation in physical activity for individuals of all ages. In 1996, *The United States Surgeon General's Report* (U.S. Surgeon General, 1996) concluded that regular physical activity has important positive effects on the musculoskeletal, cardiovascular, respiratory and endocrine systems. Furthermore, the effect of exercise on these systems is associated with a number of health benefits, including a decreased risk of premature mortality and reduced risks of coronary heart disease, hypertension, colon cancer and diabetes mellitus. In addition, regular participation in physical activity also appears to reduce depression and anxiety, improve mood and enhance our ability to perform daily tasks throughout the life span (U.S. Surgeon General, 1996).

The WHO *Guidelines for Promoting Physical Activity Among Older Persons* offer a similarly strong endorsement. The guidelines conclude that there is now compelling evidence that regular physical activity can assist in avoiding, minimizing and/or reversing many of the physical, psychological and social hazards that often accompany advancing age.

The following sections provide a brief overview of some of the physiological, psychological and social benefits of regular exercise. Whenever possible, an attempt is made to address both the acute effects of a single bout of physical activity, as well as the more persistent and long-term effects of sustained participation in exercise and physical activity. Because physical activity has been defined in many different ways, in this section, we will adopt the World Health Organization's broad and inclusive definition of physical activity, which includes all movements in everyday life, including work, recreation, exercise and sporting activities (WHO, 1997).

Table 1.1

A Summary of the Physiological Benefits of Physical Activity for Older Persons

World Health Organization, 1997

Immediate Benefits:

✓ Glucose Levels: Physical activity helps regulate blood glucose levels.

✓ Catecholamine Activity: Both adrenalin and noradrenalin levels are stimulated by physical activity.

✓ Improved Sleep: Physical activity has been shown to enhance sleep quality and quantity in individuals of all ages.

Long-term Effects:

✓ Aerobic/Cardiovascular Endurance: Substantial improvements in almost all aspects of cardiovascular functioning have been observed following appropriate physical training.

✓ Resistive Training/Muscle Strengthening: Individuals of all ages can benefit from muscle-strengthening exercises. Resistance training can have a significant impact on the maintenance of independence in old age.

✓ Flexibility: Exercise that stimulates movement throughout the range of motion assists in the preservation and restoration of flexibility.

✓ Balance/Coordination: Regular activity helps prevent and/or postpone the age-associated declines in balance and coordination that are a major risk factor for falls.

✓ Velocity of Movement: Behavioral slowing is a characteristic of advancing age. Individuals who are regularly active can often postpone these age-related declines.

The WHO Guidelines have been placed in the public domain and can be freely copied and distributed. (WHO, 1997)

Physiological Benefits of Physical Activity

The physiological benefits of participation in regular physical activity are well established (see Table 1.1). Among the short-term benefits attributed to regular exercise are improved sleep (Brassington & Hicks, 1995), improved glucose regulation (Giacca et al., 1994) and increases in catecholamine activity (Richter & Sutton, 1994). Long-term adaptation to extended exercise participation includes improved cardiovascular performance, increased muscular strength and endurance, enhanced flexibility and range of motion, decreased adiposity and improved lipid status (Spirduso, 1995). Goldberg and Hagberg (1990) suggest that the physiological responses of older adults to exercise training are essentially the same as those experienced by younger individuals. Several of the more common physiological adaptations associated with regular physical activity are discussed below.

Cardiovascular Function

Maximal oxygen consumption (VO_2max) during exercise is an excellent measure of cardiovascular fitness (McArdle, Katch & Katch, 1994). VO_2max was previously thought to decline at a constant rate with advancing age (about 10 percent per decade). This decline was considered to be relatively stable across subjects and, to a large degree, independent of physical activity status (Hodgson, 1971; Dehn & Bruce, 1972). However, a number of recent studies suggest that age-related changes in VO_2max may be more variable (Heath et al., 1981; Rogers et al., 1990). For example, highly trained individuals who maintain high activity levels often experience little or no decline in VO_2max over periods of a decade or more (Kasch, Wallace & VanCamp, 1985; Pollock et al., 1987).

Although the mechanisms by which exercise influences cardiovascular performance in older adults are complex, there is evidence to suggest that both central (increased cardiac output) and peripheral (increased oxidative capacity of the skeletal muscle) factors are involved (Hagberg & Goldberg, 1990). It is not possible to postpone age-related declines in aerobic capacity forever. Nonetheless, there is increasingly strong evidence to suggest even modest levels of physical activity can result in significant increases in cardiovascular efficiency in old age.

Pulmonary Function

Pulmonary efficiency declines with age, resulting in compromised lung elasticity and compliance (McKeown, 1965). Degenerative changes in the vertebral discs alter the shape of the thoracic cavity with a resultant reduction in pulmonary volume (McKeown, 1965). Decreased strength and mass of the thoracic muscles further compromise pulmonary efficiency (Dhar, Shastri & Lenora, 1976), as do calcification and **ossification** of the **costovertebral** and **costochondral** joints (Grant, 1972).

In young and middle-aged individuals, aerobic exercise has minimal effects on vital capacity, expiratory volumes and other measures of pulmonary performance (Shephard, 1993). However, because regular exercise is associated with reduced vertebral degeneration rates and increased thoracic muscle strength, physical activity may help preserve adequate levels of pulmonary function in older adults (Shephard, 1993). Further research is needed to determine the precise effects of exercise on pulmonary performance in older populations.

Blood Pressure

More than 20 million older Americans have hypertension (Kannel & Vokonas, 1986). While both systolic and diastolic blood pressure increase significantly with advancing age (Spirduso, 1995), several exercise-training studies have shown that physical activity can reduce systolic and diastolic blood pressure in patients with borderline hypertension (Hagberg & Goldberg, 1990). For example, Hagberg et al. (1985) demonstrated that a six-month program of low-intensity walking significantly lowered both systolic and diastolic blood pressure in hypertensive adults aged 60 to 65 years. These data suggest that exercise may have anti-hypertensive effects in older individuals similar to those previously reported in younger populations.

Blood Lipids

Aging is associated with increases in both total cholesterol and serum triglycerides (Buskirk, 1985). Hypercholesterolemia and hyperlipidemia are major medical problems that lead to the premature development of coronary artery disease (Castelli et al., 1977). Exercise training is now commonly associated with a reduction of coronary heart disease risk, and the American Heart Association (AHA) recognizes sedentary living as an independent risk factor for the development of atherosclerosis (Fletcher et al., 1992). A number of studies have shown that highly trained masters athletes exhibit favorable biochemical profiles (reduced low-density lipoprotein cholesterol, elevated high-density lipoprotein cholesterol) when compared with sedentary individuals of the same chronological age (Seals et al., 1984; Tamai et al., 1988). Because almost all instances of favorable improvements in biochemical profiles are associated with coincident decreases in body weight, it is frequently difficult to dissociate the effects of exercise from the effects of weight loss (Hagberg & Goldberg, 1990). These problems notwithstanding, there is sufficient evidence to suggest that regular exercise is associated with a decrease in body fat, which, in turn, is associated with a decrease in circulating lipids. However, the effect of exercise on blood lipids appears to be transient, and blood lipids return to pre-exercise values within a few days of cessation of physical activity (WHO, 1997).

Muscle Strength and Endurance

Muscle strength and endurance decline significantly with advancing age (Spirduso, 1995). Until recently, strength training was seldom emphasized as a component of exercise programs designed for older adults. The lifting of heavy weights requires maximal or near-maximal muscular contractions that, if incorrectly performed, can result in sharp increases in blood pressure due to a physiological mechanism known as the **Valsalva maneuver** (McArdle, Katch, & Katch, 1994). Since these acute elevations in blood pressure are potentially dangerous for hypertensive individuals, most professional organizations do not advocate strength training for older adults. However, a number of recent studies have examined the effect of dynamic strength training in elderly adults. Morgan et al. (1995) demonstrated that older adults who trained with weights for 12 months were able to gain appreciable increases in muscular strength and endurance. No adverse consequences associated with weight training were reported in this study. Fiaterone et al. (1990) demonstrated that men and women as old as 90 years can safely lift heavy weights (80 percent of 1 repetition maximum). Remarkable strength gains in excess of 100 percent were

reported for some of the muscle groups trained in this study.

Since the maintenance of adequate levels of muscular strength is critical for successfully performing many activities of daily living, exercise scientists are reevaluating the importance of strength training as a component of exercise programs for elderly adults. The American College of Sports Medicine recommends the inclusion of low- to moderate-intensity strength exercises in exercise-training regimens for older adults (ACSM, 1995).

Flexibility

Aging is associated with changes in the elasticity and compliance of connective tissue (Spirduso, 1995), resulting in significant decreases in flexibility and range of motion. Although declines in flexibility and active range of motion are observed in most seniors, there is some evidence to suggest that declines in these areas are due in part to decreased physical activity, and that not all older individuals lose flexibility at the same rate (Campanelli, 1996). Stretching exercises that emphasize range of motion and flexibility have been shown to increase ankle, knee joint and lower back flexibility in older adults (Frekany & Leslie, 1975). Almost all structured exercise programs advocate the inclusion of calisthenic exercises prior to aerobic exercise (Spirduso, 1995).

Psychological Benefits of Physical Activity

In addition to its effects on physiological variables, physical activity also can have significant psychological consequences. A summary of the long- and short-term benefits of physical activity for psychological functioning is included in Table 1.2.

Table 1.2

A Summary of the Psychological Benefits of Physical Activity for Older Persons

World Health Organization, 1997

Immediate Benefits:

✓ Relaxation: Appropriate physical activity enhances relaxation.

✓ Reduces Stress and Anxiety: There is evidence that regular physical activity can reduce stress and anxiety.

✓ Enhanced Mood State: Numerous people report elevations in mood state following appropriate physical activity.

Long-term Effects:

✓ General Well-being: Improvements in almost all aspects of psychological functioning have been observed following periods of extended physical activity.

✓ Improved Mental Health: Regular exercise can make an important contribution in the treatment of several mental illnesses, including depression and anxiety neuroses.

✓ Cognitive Improvements: Regular physical activity may help postpone age-related declines in central nervous system processing speed and improve reaction time.

✓ Motor Control and Performance: Regular activity helps prevent and/or postpone the age-associated declines in both fine and gross motor performance.

✓ Skill Acquisition: New skills can be learned and existing skills refined by all individuals regardless of age.

The WHO Guidelines have been placed in the public domain and can be freely copied and distributed. (WHO, 1997)

Among the short-term psychological benefits attributed to regular exercise are improved relaxation (Landers & Petruzzello, 1994), reduced stress and anxiety (Petruzzello et al., 1991) and improved mood state (Nieman et al., 1993). Long-term benefits include improved life satisfaction (Berger & Hecht, 1990), enhanced self-esteem and heightened self-efficacy (McAuley & Rudolph, 1995) and fewer mood state disturbances (O'Connor, Aenchbacher & Dishman, 1993). Some of the more common psychological benefits associated with regular physical activity are discussed below.

General Psychological Well-being

Although psychological health consists of both positive and negative components, previous research in the exercise sciences has focused predominantly on the effects of physical activity on negative components of psychological health, such as depression, anxiety and other stress-related disorders. McAuley and his colleagues (McAuley, 1994; McAuley & Rudolph, 1995) argued the importance of examining the relation between physical activity and more positive elements of psychological functioning, including self-esteem, self-efficacy and general well-being.

A review of 38 studies examining the relation between regular physical activity and general psychological well-being in older adult populations indicates that the vast majority of studies report a positive association between physical activity and well-being (McAuley & Rudolph, 1995). While this relationship appears to be independent of the mode of exercise employed (Mihalko & McAuley, 1996), the strength of the association is greatest for programs lasting 10 weeks or longer.

Depression and Anxiety

The incidence of depression increases significantly with age (LaRue,

Dessonville & Jarvik, 1985). However, several studies suggest that the association between chronological age and depression may be confounded by decreases in physical activity levels that usually accompany advancing age (Parent & Whall, 1986; Berkman et al., 1986). When statistical procedures are used to control for individual differences in fitness, the association between advancing age and depression is substantially reduced (Chodzko-Zajko, 1990). Accordingly, data suggesting depression increases with age may be at least partially due to the tendency for physical activity levels to decline with age and not simply due to the passage of time.

A number of studies have shown that participation in regular exercise reduces depression in patients with mild-to-moderate levels of clinical depression (Greist et al., 1979; Martinsen, Medhus & Sandvik, 1985). Similarly, studies with non-clinical populations also indicate beneficial effects of exercise on mood state and anxiety (Morgan & O'Connor, 1987). Despite this association between physical activity and depression, it has yet to be conclusively demonstrated that exercise plays a causal role in the reduction of depression (O'Connor, Aenchbacher & Dishman, 1993). Additional research is needed to examine the precise nature of the relationship between physical activity and both anxiety and depression in old age.

Cognitive Functioning

Age-related declines in **cognitive** performance are well established. However, cognition is not a unitary phenomenon and there are wide variations in the magnitude of changes in cognitive performance tasks observed with advancing age. Age-related changes in cognitive performance appear to be maximized for tasks that require rapid and complex processing, and are minimized for tasks that are more automatic or

can be performed at a self-paced rate (Chodzko-Zajko & Moore, 1994).

Despite the fact that both processing resources and cognitive performance decline with advancing age, there are often considerable differences between subjects in both the rate and extent of this decline. There is now substantial evidence to support the hypothesis that physically fit older adults often process cognitive information more efficiently than less-fit individuals of the same chronological age (Chodzko-Zajko, 1991). However, it is clear that the relationship between physical fitness and cognition is highly task-dependent. Physical fitness effects are observed more often during tasks requiring rapid cognitive processing than during self-paced or automatic processing tasks (Chodzko-Zajko & Moore, 1994). Because numerous task and subject-related factors can influence the relationship between fitness and cognition, extreme caution is warranted before making generalizations about the influence of physical fitness on cognitive performance.

Despite the presence of a cross-sectional association between fitness and cognitive performance, the effect of exercise on cognitive performance remains unclear. Several well-controlled studies successfully demonstrated improvement in cognitive performance following training (Dustman et al., 1984; Hawkins, Kramer & Capaldi; 1992; Moul, Goldman & Warren, 1995). However, at least as many studies have been unable to replicate these findings (Blumenthal et al., 1989; 1991; Panton et al., 1990). Both the magnitude of improvement in aerobic capacity and the demand-level of the cognitive task may be important factors in determining the presence or absence of training effects. It is important to point out that the magnitude of changes in cognitive performance observed following exercise training has always been small.

At present, there is no compelling evidence to suggest that short-term exercise training results in clinically significant improvements in cognition.

A number of mechanisms have been proposed to explain the relationship between physical fitness and cognitive performance in old age (Chodzko-Zajko & Moore, 1994). Some evidence suggests that highly fit adults process information in the central nervous system faster and more efficiently than less-fit individuals of the same chronological age. This increased efficiency may be secondary to improvements in cerebral circulation, nerve cell regeneration and/or changes in neurotransmitter synthesis and degradation.

Social Implications of Regular Physical Activity

The vast majority of research studies examining the effects of exercise on the aging process have focused on the physiological and psychological benefits of activity. However, it would be inappropriate to conclude this section without a brief comment about the importance of physical activity for the social functioning of older persons.

In the WHO *Guidelines for Promoting Physical Activity Among Older Persons,* a number of significant short- and long-term effects of physical activity on sociocultural variables are discussed (see Table 1.3). Empowering older individuals and assisting them in playing a more active role in society are among the social benefits attributed to physical activity.

Aging is associated with a need to adjust to changing roles. Factors such as the deaths of friends and loved ones, retirement, financial hardship, ill-health and isolation force many older people to systematically relinquish more and more of the roles that are a meaningful part of their identity (McPherson, 1990). Physical activity can help older persons better adjust to these changing roles. Activity programs provide seniors with the opportunity to widen their social networks, to stimulate new friendships and to acquire positive new roles in their retirement (McPherson, 1990, 1994).

Exercise Programming for Older Adults

Until recently, physical activity programming for older adults typically focused on a relatively small and healthy subgroup of the older adult population (Chodzko-Zajko, 1995). However, it is now clear that the beneficial effects of regular physical activity are observable in almost all older persons regardless of their physical health. Several excellent and well-publicized studies have focused attention on the benefits of regular physical activity for seniors who were previously thought to be "too old" or "too frail" to partake in structured exercise programming (Spirduso, 1995). The World Health Organization (1997) suggests that most older adults fall along a Health-Fitness Gradient, with good health and fitness at one end of the continuum, and physical frailty and dependence at the other (see Figure 1.2).

Within the WHO scheme, the physical activity needs of older persons differ substantially depending on their position along the Health-Fitness Gradient. The differing physical activity needs of the three groups are described below.

Group III: Physically Fit - Healthy

These individuals regularly engage in physical activity, are described as physically fit and healthy and have few limits in performing activities of daily living. Older adults in this group can participate in most physical activity programs, often exercising alongside individuals many years their junior.

Figure 1.2

World Health Organization Health-Fitness Gradient

	Physically Fit	*Physically Unfit*	*Physically Unfit Frail*
Healthy	GROUP III		
Unhealthy Independent		GROUP II	
Unhealthy Dependent			GROUP I

(WHO, 1997)

Group II: Physically Unfit - Unhealthy Independent

These individuals do not engage in adequate physical activity. While they still live independently in the community, they are at high risk for developing multiple chronic medical conditions that threaten their independence. Regular physical activity can help maintain independence and prevent regression into full dependency. However, physical activity programming must be individualized to account for special limitations and disabilities. *The United States Surgeon General's Report* (1996) estimates that at least 60 percent of the older adult population falls into this category.

Table 1.3

A Summary of the Social Benefits of Physical Activity for Older Persons

World Health Organization, 1997

Immediate Benefits:

✓ Empowering Older Individuals: A large proportion of the older adult population voluntarily adopts a sedentary lifestyle, which eventually threatens to reduce independence and self-sufficiency. Participation in appropriate physical activity can help empower older individuals and assist them in playing a more active role in society.

✓ Enhanced Social and Cultural Integration: Physical activity programs, particularly when carried out in small groups and/or in social environments, enhance social and intercultural interactions for many older adults.

Long-term Effects:

✓ Enhanced Integration: Regularly active individuals are less likely to withdraw from society and more likely to actively contribute to the social milieu.

✓ Formation of New Friendships: Participation in physical activity, particularly in small groups and other social environments, stimulates new friendships and acquaintances.

✓ Widened Social and Cultural Networks: Physical activity frequently provides individuals with an opportunity to widen available social networks.

✓ Role Maintenance and New Role Acquisition: A physically active lifestyle helps foster the stimulating environments necessary for maintaining an active role in society, as well as for acquiring positive new roles.

✓ Enhanced Intergenerational Activity: In many societies, physical activity is a shared activity that provides opportunities for intergenerational contact, thereby diminishing stereotypical perceptions about aging and the elderly.

The WHO Guidelines have been placed in the public domain and can be freely copied and distributed. (WHO, 1997)

Group I: Physically Unfit - Unhealthy Dependent

These individuals are no longer able to function independently in society due to a variety of physical and/or psychological reasons. Appropriate physical activity can significantly enhance the quality of life and restore independence in some areas of functioning. Physical activity programs have been developed for application in nursing homes and other residential facilities (Campanelli, 1996). A wide variety of chair and bed exercises can be performed on an individualized basis (Barry, Rich & Carlson, 1993).

Principles of Exercise Prescription for Older Adults

It is inappropriate to apply generic exercise **prescriptions** across the board for all older adults. Individual differences in health status, physical fitness and previous exercise experience require that exercise prescription be tailored to meet the specific needs of each person.

Older adults should be encouraged to seek advice from a health or exercise professional who can design a program to meet their individual needs. Previously sedentary individuals older than 40 should obtain a thorough medical examination before embarking on an exercise program (ACSM, 1995). In cases where a physician's examination is not possible, pre-exercise screening questionnaires can assist in identifying contraindications to exercise (Cardinal & Cardinal, 1995).

A large percentage of the elderly population has remained sedentary due to the mistaken belief that they were not candidates for participation in regular physical activity. While there is an extremely small number of individuals for whom exercise is medically contraindicated (Stone, 1987), the vast majority of the elderly population can benefit from participation in some form of physical activity (WHO, 1997). The emergence of specialized programs for specific clinical populations, such as cardiac rehabilitation programs, the Arthritis Foundation's PACE program and programs for diabetics, is testament to the fact that the benefits of physical activity need not be restricted to "jocks" and exercise fanatics.

The WHO *Guidelines for Promoting Physical Activity Among Older Persons* acknowledge the wide diversity of exercise regimens for older adults. Exercise, which can be an individual or group activity, can be performed in supervised or unsupervised settings. The guidelines stress that it is not necessary to have expensive facilities and equipment, and that successful programs are possible with limited resources (WHO, 1997).

The American College of Sports Medicine's *Guidelines for Exercise Testing and Prescription* (1995) notes that the general principles of exercise prescription apply to individuals of all ages. However, due to the wide range of health and fitness levels observed among seniors, special care is needed when prescribing exercise for older persons. The guidelines recognize that, for most older persons, a well-rounded exercise program consists of a cardiovascular component, resistance training and flexibility exercises. For specific exercise strategies and program design, see Chapters 5 and 6.

While recognizing the importance of individualized exercise prescription, it is possible to make some comments about general principles of exercise programming for older adults.

Activity Mode

Low-intensity, rhythmic activities that utilize large muscle groups, such as walking, jogging, bicycling and swimming, are optimal for enhancing aerobic capacity. While personal preference typically dictates the type of activity chosen, orthopedic and/or other medical factors may restrict the number of available options. An increasing number of older adults participate in other activities. such as various forms of dance and weight training. While these activities may not be appropriate for all older individuals, many people can obtain significant physiological benefits and much enjoyment from them (ACSM, 1995).

Training Frequency

To obtain a reliable training effect, two to three training sessions per week are required (ACSM, 1995). However, habitual exercisers often exercise five or six days per week without adverse consequences (ACSM, 1995). It is important to note that many of the physiological, psychological and social benefits of physical activity require regular and continuous participation and can rapidly be reversed by a return to inactivity.

Duration of Exercise

Most structured exercise programs are designed to last about 45 minutes to one hour. This time is typically divided into 15 to 20 minutes of warm-up and stretching, 20 to 30 minutes of aerobic activity and five to 10 minutes of cooldown. While this format is flexible, some evidence suggests that the aerobic component of exercise programs should last at least 20 minutes to obtain optimal cardiovascular benefits (Spirduso, 1995).

For the sedentary and frail individuals in Groups I and II of the WHO Health-Fitness Gradient, continuous activity for 45 to 60 minutes may be an unrealistic goal, at least at the onset of an exercise program. More modest exercise targets should be set for these individuals. As they slowly become re-accustomed to physical activity, exercise programs may be adjusted accordingly.

Exercise Intensity

It is a popular misconception that high-intensity exercise is required for significant physiological gain. The saying "no pain, no gain" is simply not true. Such misconceptions perpetuate inappropriate attitudes about exercise and result in large numbers of individuals avoiding potentially beneficial and enjoyable behaviors. Many older adults first learned to exercise at a time when high-intensity exercise was widely considered more effective than more modest levels of activity. In recent years there has been extensive debate regarding the utility of traditional exercise prescriptions when applied to the sedentary population (Blair, 1994). Rather than adopt a hard-and-fast stance regarding the minimum frequency, duration and intensity of exercise necessary to achieve a training effect, individuals should be encouraged to simply increase their activity level without setting rigid (and frequently intimidating) exercise prescriptions.

Conclusion

Advancing age is characterized by a progressive and insidious decline in the functional capacity of most physiological systems. While these declines in functional capacity are, to a large extent, inevitable and inescapable, considerable differences exist between individuals in the rate and extent of this decline. Several lines of research suggest that individuals who engage in healthful behaviors can often postpone or reduce these adverse consequences and, thus, deviate from expected patterns of aging.

The United States Surgeon General's Report on Physical Activity and Health recommends incorporating regular physical activity, which has significant physiological, psychological and socio-cultural benefits, into the everyday lives of all Americans of all ages. The World Health Organization (WHO, 1997) concludes that there is now ample evidence that physical activity is associated with improvements in functional ability and health status and may frequently prevent or diminish the severity of certain diseases.

The benefits of physical activity are not restricted to the healthiest segment of the older-adult population. On the contrary, there are significant benefits of physical activity for even the most frail members of society. As the advantages of physical activity for older adults become more widely appreciated, it is likely that a growing proportion of the population, regardless of age, will begin to include exercise as an integral component of their everyday routine.

References

American College of Sports Medicine. (1995). *Guidelines for Exercise Testing and Prescription.* (5th ed.) Baltimore: Williams & Wilkins.

Arking, R. (1991). *Biology of Aging: Observations and Principles.* Englewood Cliffs, N.J.: Prentice-Hall, Inc.

Baker, G.T. & Martin, G.R. (1994). Biological aging and longevity: Underlying mechanisms and potential intervention strategies. *Journal of Aging and Physical Activity,* 2, 4, 304-328.

Balin, A.K. (1994). *Practical Handbook of Human Biologic Age Determination.* Boca Raton, Fla.: CRC Press.

Balin, A.K. (1983). Testing the free radical theory of aging. In R.C. Adelman & G.S. Roth (Eds.) *Testing the Theories of Aging.* Boca Raton, Fla.: CRC Press.

Barry, H., Rich, B. & Carlson, T. (1993). How exercise can benefit older patients: A practical approach. *The Physician and Sportsmedicine,* 21, 2, 124-140.

Berger, B.G. & Hecht, L.M (1990). Exercise, aging and psychological well-being: The mind-body question. In A.C. Ostrow (Ed.) *Aging and Motor Behavior* (307-323). Indianapolis: Benchmark Press.

Berkman, L.F., Berkman, C.S., Kasl, S., Leo, D.H., Ostfeld, A.M., Coroni-Huntley, J. & Brody, J. (1986). Depressive symptoms in relation to physical health and functioning in the elderly. *American Journal of Epidemiology,* 124, 372-388.

Birren, J.E. (1959). Principles of research on aging. In J.E. Birren (Ed.) *Handbook of Aging and the Individual* (3-32). Chicago, Ill.: University of Chicago Press.

Bjorksten, J. (1968). The cross linkage theory of aging. *Journal of the American Geriatric Society,* 16, 408-427.

Blair, S.N. (1994). Physical activity, fitness, and coronary heart disease. In C. Bouchard, R.J. Shephard, T. Stephens (Eds.) *Physical Activity, Fitness, and Health.* Champaign, Ill.: Human Kinetics.

Blumenthal, J.A., Emery, C.F., Madden, D.J., et al. (1991). Long-term effects of exercise on psychological functioning in older men and women. *Journal of Gerontology,* 46, 352-361.

Blumenthal, J.A., Emery, C.F., Madden, D.J., et al. (1989). Cardiovascular and behavioral effects of aerobic exercise training in healthy older men and women. *Journal of Gerontology,* 44, 147-157.

Bokovy, J.L. & Blair, S.N. (1994). Aging and exercise and health perspective. *Journal of Aging and Physical Activity,* 2, 3, 243-260.

Brassington, G.S. & Hicks, R.A. (1995). Aerobic exercise and self-reported sleep quality in elderly individuals. *Journal of Aging and Physical Activity,* 3, 2, 120-134.

Buskirk, E.R. (1985). Health Maintenance and Longevity: Exercise. In E.L. Schneider et al., (Ed.) *The Handbook of the Biology of Aging.* (2nd ed.) New York: Van Nostrand Reinhold.

Campanelli, L.C. (1996). Mobility changes in older adults: Implications for practitioners. *Journal of Aging and Physical Activity,* 4, 2, 105-118.

Cardinal, B.J. & Cardinal, M.K. (1995). Screening efficiency of the revised physical activity readiness questionnaire in older adults. *Journal of Aging and Physical Activity,* 3, 3, 299-308.

Castelli, W.P., Doyle, J.T., Gordon, T., Hames, C.G., Hjortland, M.C., Hulley, S.B., Kagan, A. & Zukel, W.J. (1977). HDL cholesterol and other lipids in coronary heart disease: The Cooperative Lipoprotein Phenotyping Study. *Circulation,* 55, 767-772.

Chodzko-Zajko, W.J. (1995). Editorial: Addressing the physical activity needs of the physically frail and the oldest old. *Journal of Aging and Physical Activity,* 3, 3, 221-222.

Chodzko-Zajko, W.J. (1994). A multivariate approach to the quantification of biologic age. In Balin, A.K. (Ed.) *Practical Handbook of Human Biologic Age Determination* (157-171). New York: CRC Press.

Chodzko-Zajko, W.J. (1993). Editorial: Great beginnings for JAPA. *Journal of Aging and Physical Activity,* 1, 1, 1.

Chodzko-Zajko, W.J. (1991). Physical fitness, cognitive performance and aging. *Medicine and Science in Sports and Exercise,* 23, 868-872.

Chodzko-Zajko, W.J. (1990). The influence of general health status on the relationship between chronological age and depressed mood state. *Journal of Geriatric Psychiatry,* 23, 13-22.

Chodzko-Zajko, W.J. & Moore, K.A. (1994). Physical fitness and cognitive functioning in aging. *Exercise and Sport Science Reviews,* 22, 195-220.

Chodzko-Zajko, W.J. & Ringel, R.L. (1987). Physiological fitness measures and sensory and motor performance in aging. *Experimental Gerontology,* 22, 5, 317-328.

Comroe, J.H. (1965). *Physiology of Respiration.* Chicago, Ill.: Year Book Medical Publishers.

Cousins, S.O. (1997). Elderly tomboys: Sources of self-efficacy for physical activity in late life. *Journal of Aging and Physical Activity,* 5, 2, in press.

Cousins, S.O. & Vertinsky, P.A. (1995). Recapturing the physical activity experiences of the old: A study of three women. *Journal of Aging and Physical Activity,* 3, 2, 146-162.

Dehn, M.M. & Bruce, R.A. (1972). Longitudinal variations in maximal oxygen intake with age and activity. *Journal of Applied Physiology,* 33, 6, 805-807.

Dhar, S., Shastri, S.R. & Lenora, R.A.K. (1976). Aging and the respiratory system. *Medical Clinics of North America,* 60, 1121-1139.

Dustman, R.E., Ruhling, R.O., Russell, E.M., Shearer, D.E., Bonekat, H.W., Shigeoka, J.W., Wood, J.S. & Bradford, D.C. (1984). Aerobic exercise training and improved neuropsychological function of older individuals. *Neurobiology of Aging,* 5, 35-42.

Fiaterone, M.A., Marks, E.C., Ryan, N.D., Meredith, C.N., Lipsitz, L.A. & Evans, W.J. (1990). High-intensity strength training in nonagenarians. *Journal of the American Medical Association,* 263, 3029-3024.

Fletcher, G.F., Blair, S.N., Blumenthal, J., Caspersen, C., Chaitman, B., Epstein, S., Falls, H., Sivarajan-Froelicher, E.S., Froelicher, V.F. & Pina, I.L. (1992). Statement on exercise: Benefits and recommendations for physical activity programs for all Americans. A statement for health professionals by the Committee on Exercise and Cardiac Rehabilitation of the Council on Clinical Cardiology, American Heart Association. *Circulation,* 86, 340-344.

Fowles D.G. (1991). The numbers game: Pyramid power. *Aging,* 2, 58-59.

Frekany, G.A. & Leslie, D.K. (1975). Effects of an exercise program on selected flexibility measurements of senior citizens. *Gerontologist,* 15, 182-183.

Fries J.F. & Crapo L.M. (1981). *Vitality and Aging.* San Francisco: Freeman.

Gerber J. (1989). *Lifetrends.* New York: Macmillan Publishing Co.

Giacca, A., Shi, Z.Q., Marliss, E.B., Zinman, B. & Vranic, M. (1994). Physical activity, fitness, and Type I diabetes. In C. Bouchard, R.J. Shephard & T. Stephens (Eds.) *Physical Activity, Fitness and Health: International Proceedings and Consensus Statement* (656-668). Champaign, Ill.: Human Kinetics.

Goldberg, A.P. & Hagberg, J.M. (1990). Physical exercise and the elderly. In: E.L. Schneider & J.W. Rowe (Eds.) *Handbook of the Biology of Aging* (407-423). San Diego: Academic Press.

Grant, J.C.B. (1972). *Grant's Atlas of Anatomy.* Baltimore: Williams and Wilkins.

Greist, J.H., Klein, M.H., Eischens, R.R., Farris, J., Gurman, A.S. & Morgan, W.P. (1979). Running as a treatment for depression. *Comprehensive Psychiatry,* 20, 41-54.

Hagberg, J.M., Allen, W.K., Seals, D.R., Hurley, B.F., Ehasani, A.A. & Holloszy, J.O. (1985). A hemodynamic comparison of young and older endurance athletes during exercise. *Journal of Applied Physiology,* 58, 2041-6.

Harman, D. (1956). Aging: A theory based on free radical and radiation chemistry. *Journal of Gerontology,* 11, 298-300.

Hawkins, H., Kramer, A.F & Capaldi, D. (1992). Aging, exercise, and attention. *Psychology and Aging,* 7, 643-653.

Hayflick, L. (1985). Theories of biological aging. *Experimental Gerontology,* 20, 145-159.

Hayflick, L. (1965). The limited in vitro lifespan of human diploid cell strains. *Experimental Cellular Respiration,* 37, 614-635.

Heath, G.W., Hagberg, J.M., Ehasani, A.A. & Holloszy, J.O. (1981). A physiological comparison of young and older endurance athletes during exercise. *Journal of Applied Physiology,* 58, 6, 2041-2046.

Heikkinen, E., Suominen, H., Era, P. & Lyyra, A.L. (1994). Variations in aging parameters, their sources, and possibilities of predicting physiological age. In A.K. Balin (Ed.) *Practical Handbook of Human Biologic Age Determination* (71-92). New York: CRC Press.

Hodgson, J.L. (1971). Age and aerobic capacity of urban midwestern males. Ph.D. Dissertation, University of Minnesota.

Jones, C.J. & Rikli, R.E. (1994). The revolution in aging: Implications for curriculum development and professional preparation in physical education. *Journal of Aging and Physical Activity,* 2, 3, 261-272.

Kallman, F.J. & Sander, G. (1948). Twin studies on aging and longevity. *Journal of Heredity,* 39, 349-357.

Kannel, W.B. & Vokonas, P.S. (1986). Primary risk factors for coronary heart disease in the elderly: The Framingham Study. In N.K. Wenger & C.D. Furburg (Eds.) *Current Heart Disease in the Elderly* (60-95). London: Elsevier.

Kasch, F.W., Boyer, J.L., Van Camp, S.P., Verity, L.S. & Wallace, J.P. (1990). The effects of physical activity and inactivity on aerobic power in older men: A longitudinal study. *The Physician and Sportsmedicine,* 18, 73-83.

Kasch, F.W., Wallace, J.P. & VanCamp, S.P. (1985). Effects of 18 years endurance exercise on the physical work capacity of older men. *Journal of Cardiopulmonary Rehabilitation,* 5, 308-312.

Kim, H.S. & Tanaka, K. (1995). The assessment of functional age using Activities of Daily Living Performance Tests: A study of Korean women. *Journal of Aging and Physical Activity,* 3, 1, 39-48.

Lakatta, E.G. (1990). Changes in cardiovascular function with aging. *European Heart Journal,* 11, 22-29.

Landers, D.M. & Petruzzello, S.J. (1994). Physical activity, fitness, and anxiety. In C. Bouchard, R.J. Shephard & T. Stephens (Eds.) *Physical Activity, Fitness and Health: International Proceedings and Consensus Statement* (868-882). Champaign, Ill.: Human Kinetics.

LaRue, A., Dessonville, C. & Jarvik, L.F. (1985). Aging and Mental Disorders. In J.E. Birren & K.W. Schaie (Eds.) *Handbook of the Psychology of Aging.* New York: Van Nostrand Reinhold.

Martinsen, E.W., Medhus, A. & Sandvik, L. (1985). Effects of aerobic exercise on depression: A controlled study. *British Medical Journal,* 291, 109.

McArdle, W.D., Katch, F.I. & Katch, V.L. (1994). *Essentials of Exercise Physiology.* Philadelphia: Lea & Febiger.

McAuley, E. (1994). Physical activity and psychosocial outcomes. In C. Bouchard, R.J. Shephard & T. Stephens (Eds.) *Physical Activity, Fitness and Health: International Proceedings and Consensus Statement* (551-568). Champaign, Ill.: Human Kinetics.

McAuley, E. & Rudolph, D. (1995). Physical activity, aging, and psychological well-being. *Journal of Aging and Physical Activity,* 3, 1, 67-98.

McGrath, J.E. & Kelly, J.R. (1985). *Time and Human Interaction: Toward a Social Psychology of Time.* New York: Guildford.

McKeown, F. (1965). *Pathology of the Aged.* London: Butterworths.

McPherson, B.D. (1994). Sociocultural perspectives on aging and physical activity. *Journal of Aging and Physical Activity,* 2, 4, 329-353.

McPherson, B.D. (1990). *Aging as a Social Process*. Toronto: Butterworths.

Medvedev, Z.A. (1981). Age changes and the rejuvenation processes related to reproduction. *Mech Aging Dev*, 17, 331-359.

Mihalko, S.L. & McAuley, E. (1996). Strength training effects on subjective well-being and physical function in the elderly. *Journal of Aging and Physical Activity*, 4, 1, 56-68.

Morgan, A.L., Ellison, J.D., Chandler, M.P. & Chodzko-Zajko, W.J. (1995). The supplemental benefits of strength training for aerobically active postmenopausal women. *Journal of Aging and Physical Activity*, 3, 332-339.

Morgan, W.P. & O'Connor, P.J. (1987). Exercise and mental health. In R.K. Dishman (Ed.) *Exercise Adherence* (91-121). Champaign, Ill.: Human Kinetics.

Moul, J.L., Goldman, B. & Warren, B. (1995). Physical activity and cognitive performance in the older population. *Journal of Aging and Physical Activity*, 3, 2, 135-144.

Nieman, D.C., Warren, B.J., Dotson, R.G., Butterworth, D.E. & Henson, D.A. (1993). Physical activity, psychological well-being, and mood state in elderly women. *Journal of Aging and Physical Activity*, 1, 1, 22-33.

O'Connor, P.J., Aenchbacher, L.E. & Dishman, R.K. (1993). Physical activity and depression in the elderly. *Journal of Aging and Physical Activity*, 1, 1, 34-58.

Panton, L.B., Graves, J.E., Pollock, M.L., Hagberg, J.M. & Chen, W. (1990). Effect of aerobic resistance training on fractionated reaction time and speed of movement. *Journal of Gerontology*, 45, 26-31.

Parent, C.J. & Whall, A.L. (1986). Are physical activity, self-esteem and depression related? *Journal of Geriatric Nursing*, 10, 8-11.

Partridge, S.M. (1970). Biological role of cutaneous elastin. In W. Montagna, J.P. Bentley & R.L. Dobson (Eds.) *Advances in Biology of Skin* (69-87). New York: Meredith.

Petruzzello, S.J., Landers, D.M., Hatfield, B.D., Kubitz, K.A. & Salazar, W. (1991). A meta-analysis on the anxiety reducing effects of acute and chronic exercise. *Sports Medicine*, 11, 143-182.

Pollock, M.L., Foster, C., Knapp, D., Rod, J.L. & Schmidt, D.H. (1987). Effect of age and training on aerobic capacity and body composition of masters athletes. *Journal of Applied Physiology*, 62, 725-731.

Richter, E.A. & Sutton, J.A. (1994). Hormonal adaptations to physical activity. In C. Bouchard, R.J. Shephard & T. Stephens (Eds.) *Physical Activity, Fitness and Health: International Proceedings and Consensus Statement* (331-342). Champaign, Ill.: Human Kinetics.

Rogers, M.A., Hagberg, J.M., Martin, W.H. & Holloszy, J.O. (1990). Decline in VO$_2$max with aging in master athletes and sedentary men. *Journal of Applied Physiology*, 68, 5, 2195-2199.

Rose, C.L. (1972). The measurement of social age. *Aging and Human Development*, 3, 153-168.

Schroots, J.J. & Birren, J.E. (1990). Concepts of time and aging in science. In J.E. Birren & K.W. Schaie (Eds.) *The Handbook of the Psychology of Aging* (3rd ed.) (45-66). San Diego: Academic Press.

Seals, D.R., Allen, W.K., Hurley, B.F., Dalsky, G.P., Ehasani, A.A. & Hagberg, J.M. (1984). Elevated high-density lipoprotein levels in older endurance athletes. *American Journal of Cardiology*, 54, 390-393.

Shephard, R.J. (1993). Aging respiratory function and exercise. *Journal of Aging and Physical Activity*, 1, 1, 59-83.

Spirduso, W.W. (1995). *Physical Dimensions of Aging*. Champaign, Ill.: Human Kinetics.

Stone, W.J. (1987). *Adult Fitness Programs*. Glenview, Ill.: Scott Foresman.

Tomai, T., Nakai, T., Hirotoda, T., Fujiwara, R., Miyabo, S., Higuchi, M. & Kobayashi, S. (1988). *Journal of Gerontology: Medical Sciences*, 43, 4, 75-79.

U.S. Census Bureau. (1990). Projections of the population of the United States by age, sex and race: 1983-2080. Current

Population Reports, Series P-25. Washington D.C.: U.S. Govt. Printing Office.

U.S. Surgeon General's Report. (1996). *Physical Activity and Health*. Washington D.C.: U.S. Government Printing Office.

Vandervoort, A.A., Chesworth, B.M., Cunningham, D.A., Paterson, D.H., Rechnitzer, P.A. & Koval, J.J. (1992). Age and sex effects on the mobility of the human ankle. *Journal of Gerontology: Medical Sciences,* 47, M17-M24.

Walford, R.L. (1987). MHC regulation of aging: An extension of the immunologic theory of aging. In H.R. Warner et al. (Eds.) *Modern Biological Theories of Aging*. New York: Raven Press.

Walford, R.L. (1983). Supergenes: Histocompatibility, immunologic and other parameters in aging. In W. Regelson & F.M. Sinex (Eds.) *Intervention in the Aging Process, Part B: Basic Research and Preclinical Screening*. New York: Alan R. Liss.

World Health Organization. (1997). The Heidelberg Guidelines for Promoting Physical Activity Among Older Persons. *Journal of Aging and Physical Activity,* 5, 1, 2-8.

Zopf, P.E. (1986). *America's Older Population*. Houston, Texas: Cap and Gown Press, Inc.

CHAPTER TWO

understanding and motivating

OLDER ADULTS

Sheri Thompson & Susan J. Hoekenga

Sheri Thompson, M.A., is a clinical psychology doctoral candidate at the California School of Professional Psychology in San Diego. She specializes in the application of cognitive and behavioral principles for making health-related changes, such as increasing physical activity and improving dietary habits. She has developed curriculum and trained physical activity counselors for Project GRAD (Graduate Ready for Activity Daily), and designed and supervised telephone counseling and mail follow-up for Project GRAD participants. She currently works at San Diego State University with Project PACE (Patient-centered Assessment and Counseling for Exercise), which offers training and materials that enable healthcare providers to briefly assess and effectively counsel their patients about making physical activity and dietary changes.

Susan J. Hoekenga, M.P.A., M.S.G., has worked in the field of aging for 20 years. She has been involved with aging policy issues at the federal, state and local level, and is currently building programs to reach under-served, frail and low-income elders for a non-profit agency. Hoekenga completed her graduate degrees in public administration and gerontology at the University of Southern California in 1995.

How does a fitness instructor learn to address individual needs and facilitate positive changes in health and fitness behaviors? This can be a difficult task, especially when the instructor's viewpoint differs from those of their clients. Your professional role extends beyond the scope of technical instruction and demonstrating proper form for a stretch or the operation of strength-training equipment. Health behaviors such as exercise are simply one aspect of a complex life, so attempts to promote health-behavior changes must take into account the individual's unique lifestyle. While competent technical instruction is crucial, fitness professionals also must collaborate with each client to develop and implement a fitness program that complements the individual's objectives, personality and life demands.

The ability to adapt your work to the differing needs of each client is particularly important when working with older adults because, as you will learn, diversity is the theme that best characterizes this population. Imagine trying to describe all 30-year-olds in a few sentences. You probably would be quick to note vast differences between people of that age group. Why would we expect those same diverse individuals to become more similar to one another by the time they reach their senior years? Older Americans vary widely in terms of physical and psychological health, cultural and ethnic backgrounds, economic means, living conditions, availability of social support, perspectives on aging and physical activity, and just about every other aspect of life!

Individuals of similar ages do share some common ground as they have gone through some of the same historical events and life experiences. It is important to learn about issues and viewpoints commonly shared by older adults. A basic understanding of the aging process can help you listen for and understand common themes that may emerge. With these issues in mind, you can apply sound behavior-change principles to promote positive, sustainable gains in your clients' fitness and health. This chapter covers common issues related to aging, as well as specific behavior-change, leadership and communication strategies to use while working with older adults. Combined with your fitness expertise, this knowledge of the aging process and recommended strategies will enable you to better serve your older clients.

SOCIETY'S IMAGE OF OLDER ADULTS

Media Characterization of Older Adults

The media has done much to shape our image of aging. There are many negative stereotypes associated with growing older and, until recently, older persons often have been stereotyped as unproductive, unhealthy and uninteresting people who are simply waiting to die. In accordance with these stereotypes, the popular arts and media have frequently portrayed older people as ill, senile, isolated and even institutionalized. These stereotypes have led to a long-standing emphasis on the losses and physical declines related to aging. In reality, only 4 percent of those over age 65 and 17 percent of those over age 85 live in institutions (Ferrini & Ferrini, 1993). In 1981, 60 percent of adults over age 65 used less than $100 worth of acute Medicare-reimbursed services, and only one in five seniors indicated they were debilitated by health problems (Davis, 1986). Many older adults —even seniors with chronic or long-term conditions such as osteoporosis, diabetes, vascular disease and cataracts —are interested in preserving their health. The vast majority of seniors want to remain as self-sufficient as possible by keeping their minds and bodies in shape. You play a major role in this process by providing them with a means to do so.

Researchers' Perspectives on Older Adults

Unfortunately, early theories on aging may have contributed to negative stereotypes by suggesting that aging was a "problem" that needed to be explained sociologically. One of the first explanations offered on the aging process suggested that a mutual withdrawal occurs between older people and society. Based on a study of older Kansas City housing-project residents in the late 1950s, researchers suggested that older people withdraw from the world around them due to an awareness of their diminishing capacities and the short time they have left to live. According to the theory, at the same time this occurs, society disengages from the elderly to make room for younger adults. The Disengagement Theory has been abandoned primarily because it emphasizes decline and loss as inevitable without offering an adequate explanation for the tremendous variation among older adults.

Many older adults adapt well to losses and remain engaged in relationships with others and in living life to the fullest. Recent research has focused on emotional development across the life span. A popular current theory, called the Socioemotional Selectivity Theory (SST), defines successful aging as one's ability to develop and maintain a sense of well-being (Carstensen & Turk-Charles, 1994). According to this theory, emotionally mature adults focus on their strengths, and adapt to changes that occur over the life span in ways that maintain or enhance life satisfaction. Aging itself does not ensure emotional maturity and enhanced life satisfaction; rather, these qualities result from one's ability to foster their development. For example, older adults often have smaller social networks than younger adults. Though older people who are aging successfully have less frequent social contacts, those they do have are characterized by stronger emotional relationships. In this case, adaptation occurs by emphasizing quality over quantity of friends.

Because life satisfaction is affected by personal preferences and needs, the Socioemotional Selectivity model has some important implications for exercise programs. First, in addition to desired health and fitness benefits, fitness professionals should be sensitive to possible life-satisfaction needs. For example, a senior with numerous social connections who primarily desires a personal physical challenge may enjoy solitary pursuits like walking or swimming. Some older clients may appreciate the opportunities for social contact, in addition to the health benefits derived from exercise. For these people, group activities, such as weight-training classes, basketball or aerobics may be the most appropriate mode of activity. Additionally, focus on what seniors can do, rather than over-emphasizing limitations or disabilities.

Impact of Negative Stereotypes on Exercise Programs for Older Adults

Stereotypes are problematic because they restrict our ways of seeing and interacting with members of the stereotyped groups. Steuart (1993) noted that programs based upon stereotypes focus on a small subset of the intended population, and neglect the priorities and needs of others in the group. For example, exercise programs designed for extremely frail elders cannot meet the needs of all older adults because they may neglect those of healthy, fit seniors.

Older adults are aware of society's stereotypes, including the expectation that they "act their age." They receive messages about the acceptability of physical activity, including the beliefs that growing older should go hand in hand with decreased physical activity, and older adults should slow down and "take it easy." People who believe that exercise is inappropriate or unnatural for older adults will not be inclined to develop or support exercise programming for this group, restricting the scope of exercise options for those who are motivated to be physically active.

Additionally, there is a prevalent stereotype that senior citizens are unmotivated or incapable of helping themselves. Some people also subscribe to the false notion that older adults become overly preoccupied with their own personal concerns. Both of these stereotypes contradict the real need to develop programs that actively involve elders in health-promoting activities. They also overlook older adults' ability to engage in activities that benefit themselves and others in society.

Unfortunately, stereotyping also has led many health professionals and the public in general to view the elderly as less worthy of investment than the young. There is a temptation to encourage older persons to tolerate even reversible conditions rather than take a proactive approach to their well-being. Such treatment may convey the message that seniors should adjust to the circumstances of their lives without actively attempting to alter them (Steuart, 1993). Only recently has there begun to be an appreciation for the value of developing and promoting physical activity programs for older adults.

UNDERSTANDING YOUR OLDER CLIENTS: IMPORTANT ISSUES IN LATER LIFE

Responsibilities to Others

Today, nearly 80 percent of all caregiving responsibilities are carried out by families (Cantor, 1991). As the health and functional status of the elderly declines, there is a growing reliance on spouses, children and siblings for assistance. Needs range from relatively minor assistance with transportation, shopping and help with yard maintenance, to the need for crucial tasks such as bathing and personal grooming. In many cases, the primary caregivers themselves are 65 and older. Because nearly 90 percent of all caregivers are women (Cantor, 1991), older women will continue to face increasing caregiver responsibilities.

Psychological Issues Associated with Aging

Because aging often is associated with loss (e.g., loss of friends, health,

income, career), there has been a great deal of interest in whether older people are more likely to suffer from mental health problems, such as loneliness, anxiety and depression, than other age groups. As a whole, the elderly are no more likely to be anxious or depressed than any other age group (Ferrini & Ferrini, 1993). However, depression is the mental health problem most frequently identified by older clients who report psychological distress. One study found that more than 10 percent of community-dwelling elders reported feeling ill at ease or sad (Kane et al., 1989). In addition to biological influences, major life changes and recurring losses also can lead to increased depression and/or anxiety for some older adults.

Personality and Aging

Research clearly suggests that personality characteristics are relatively stable over time (Kogan, 1990). In fact, during old age, you "become more like you initially were." If an individual tended to be cranky, negative, worried or unpleasant as an adult, they will carry those same traits into old age. Warm and generous adults tend to be warm and generous elders.

This is not to suggest that an individual's personality stays the same over time. Personality changes do occur, but they tend to result from life experiences—not aging per se (Kogan, 1990). Throughout their life, every person has a unique set of experiences—some positive and some negative. Events such as the birth of a child, the death of a friend, a car accident, and moving to a new home all are important episodes that shape overall levels of life satisfaction. The longer people live, the more experiences influence the way they view the world and relate to others.

Cognitive Functioning in Later Life: Intelligence and Learning Ability

Contrary to popular belief, intelligence is not a single aptitude. It actually is composed of a number of abilities, and while crystallized intelligence, or knowledge accumulated over the life span (through education, work experiences, reading, etc.), generally remains stable over time, older adults do experience some declines in fluid intelligence, such as impromptu reasoning and problem-solving abilities (Salthouse, 1991). Research also has suggested that though older adults are quite capable of learning, the speed of learning and of processing new information may decline with age (Salthouse, 1991; Spotts & Schewe, 1989). As with all characteristics of older adults, there is tremendous variation in the effects of aging upon these abilities.

The Effects of Age-related Physical Changes on Motivation to Exercise

Although people age at the same chronological rate, self-perceptions do not automatically correspond to a particular physical age. In addition to physical status, lifestyle choices and experiences affect age-related self-perception. At age 75, a person who is physically strong, content with relationships, and practices healthy eating and exercise habits may feel 55 or 60. Another 75-year-old who suffers from arthritis, feels lonely much of the time, is obese and smokes cigarettes may feel like a 90-year-old.

In Chapter 1 you learned that normal changes occur as a person grows older. There is a gradual decline in some of our maximum functional capacities beginning in our 20s and 30s. When it begins, the decline is barely perceptible, but over time there are decreases in reaction time and an overall decline in organ function (Kane et al., 1989). In general, older people experience a lower tolerance for physical stress than younger adults. As declines become cumulative, older adults begin to notice the changes. They feel their age "beginning to creep up on them." The cumulative effects of unhealthy lifestyle choices (e.g., poor eating habits, smoking, alcohol abuse, etc.) make typical declines even more pronounced.

Older adults may not change health-related behaviors in response to physical declines until a critical level is reached (Kane et al., 1989). Once noticed, physical declines may trigger a fear of lost independence centering around losing the ability to get around easily, losing intelligence and memory-related functions, and losing good health. Some sedentary seniors simply accept decreased physical abilities, remain non-active, and even continue unhealthy habits such as cigarette smoking and eating high-fat foods. Lifelong exercisers who have a stroke, acute illness or an accident may become newly concerned about physically exerting themselves, thinking that exercise caused the condition or did nothing to prevent it. Under these circumstances, individuals may reduce their activity level because they believe that exercise can be harmful (or not beneficial).

In contrast, other older adults will want to address age-related declines directly by beginning or modifying an exercise routine. Examples of this include seniors who begin exercising after a stroke, fall, illness, doctor's order or another event that makes them aware of their own (or a peer's) declining physical condition. Regular exercisers who experience performance declines may become determined to work harder in their current physical activity program. Such individuals also may combine healthy exercise behaviors with other positive changes, such as increased compliance with prescription medications and eating a balanced, nutritious diet.

OLDER ADULTS MOST LIKELY TO SEEK EXERCISE GUIDANCE

The "age wave" sweeping America is a heterogeneous lot—wealthy and poor, young-old and old-old, healthy and those with chronic ailments. There are probably more dissimilarities among the elderly than there are common traits. These differences significantly impact the profile of older persons who typically seek out formal exercise programs, and are most evident when viewed by gender, ethnicity and income.

Demographic factors associated with lower participation rates in physical activity programs include low income, being a member of an ethnic minority and being older than 85 with multiple health problems. For low-income and minority seniors in particular, the biggest deterrents are lack of access to exercise programs and lack of knowledge about the benefits of exercise for older adults. These seniors also may not be aware of (or have access to) financial and community resources that enable them to practice healthy habits such as proper nutrition and preventive healthcare.

Not surprisingly, health status also is strongly associated with income, education and social class; people with higher incomes and education levels tend to be healthier. They are more likely to be aware of the benefits of exercise and able to manage the expense of fitness facility memberships, exercise equipment, transportation to program sites, etc. There is little research on the characteristics of older adults most likely to seek physical activity assistance. However, unless you work for a program or

A Comparison of Elders

There is a growing appreciation for the idea that everyone does not age in the same way or at the same rate. As we try to understand aging, it is essential to keep in mind the principle of individual variation. Let's briefly look at three sub-groups of the older-adult population (Ferrini & Ferrini, 1993).

Community Dwelling Elders. Ninety-five percent of people age 65 or older reside in the community. Although seniors experience more chronic conditions and impairments than middle-age adults, most report generally good health. Those most likely to need help are the very old, or those over age 85.

Nursing Home Residents. While only 5 percent of elders live in nursing homes at any given time, nearly 20 percent of people over the age of 85 will be admitted to a nursing home. Among elderly nursinghome residents there are two distinct populations: One group leaves fairly quickly (three to six months), while the other group stays several years. Long-term patients tend to be older and have both physical and mental diagnoses. About one-third of nursing home discharges go back to the community.

Physically Active Elders. The number of older adults who regularly exercise has increased dramatically within the last few decades. Large-scale studies find between 8 percent and 33 percent of seniors engage in regular physical activity that enables them to maintain or improve cardiorespiratory fitness. Other seniors exercise regularly enough to gain health benefits, but perform at intensities too low for cardiovascular fitness benefits.

facility serving many minority or low-income clients, those most likely to seek your exercise consultation will be Caucasian, from middle- to upper-level economic and educational backgrounds. This is similar to the profile of younger and middle-aged adult health club members.

Among both non-white and white populations, women live significantly longer than men. The life expectancy of Caucasians is about 73 years for men and nearly 80 years for women (Himes, 1992). By age 80, there are two females for every living male (Myers, 1990). Because life expectancy is greater for women than for men, exercise programs will continue to be needed by more older women than men, particularly those older than 75.

Meeting the Needs of a Diverse Older Adult Population

Adults who are over the age of 65 today grew up during the Depression and World War II, when money was often tight and work was physically strenuous. Many seniors performed labor-intensive activities in the military, while doing household chores or on the job. Exercise was a part of daily life, not a health benefit in and of itself. As younger adults, many of these seniors simply may have lacked the time, money or interest to engage in a formal fitness program.

Now, a growing range of seniors have recognized the benefits of voluntary physical activity, and exercise programs must be developed to address their needs and encourage increased participation in formal exercise programs. Effective exercise promotion for older adults should include the following elements:

✓ consideration of the exercise attitudes and behaviors of each individual

✓ explanation of the risks and complications of exercise

✓ a medical assessment to determine fitness level

✓ exercise prescriptions tailored to each individual

✓ monitored effects of exercise

✓ use of motivational tools to increase compliance

✓ if necessary, reference to other professionals for nutritional evaluation or counseling

The use of these actions will ensure that the programs you design with and for older adults will meet their needs, despite individual differences.

THE FUNCTIONS OF EXERCISE FOR OLDER ADULTS

Exercise to Improve or Maintain Fitness or Health

How can you help older people improve physically when their functional capacity is declining? Typically there is plenty of room for improvement as most adults have never operated at their maximum ability in any area. Consider the analogy of an automobile that can be driven 100 miles per hour. Despite this capacity for speed, its driver usually drives between 25 and 60 miles per hour because that is as fast as they need to go. Even after the car has aged, and "wear and tear" have reduced the engine's former potential for speed, the car is still quite capable of performing at speeds far greater than those normally used by its driver. Similarly, most older adults can develop their physical abilities beyond current levels. By adopting and adhering to a regular exercise program, your older clients can improve their functional capacity by increasing current muscle strength, flexibility and aerobic endurance.

It also is true that a properly maintained automobile that has been driven at reasonable speeds can perform well for much longer than a poorly maintained car that was pushed beyond reasonable limits. Older adults can likewise develop good maintenance habits (exercise and health practices) to sustain their health well into advanced age. Cars driven regularly also tend to remain in better condition than cars left unused for years. Physical capabilities are similar; to maintain or improve a skill or function, it must be utilized. Exercise programs for seniors can improve or maintain current physical capabilities, and can even lead to a positive self image, better sleep, decreased blood pressure and assistance with weight control (Ferrini & Ferrini, 1993).

Exercise to Improve Mental and Emotional Status

Research on the psychological benefits of physical activity varies widely in terms of methodology, quality and generalizability (Brown, 1992). Older exercisers tend to believe they are more in control of their own lives than older non-exercisers, and this sense of personal control is a significant factor in warding off depression (Ferrini & Ferrini, 1993). Numerous psychosocial benefits of exercise for older adults also have been reported, including improved self-esteem, self-confidence and sense of pride; decreased stress and insomnia symptoms; a socially appropriate outlet for anger; decreased dependent behaviors; improved socialization; and an increased sense of life purpose (Brown, 1990; Burlew, Jones & Emerson, 1991; Sonstroem & Morgan, 1989; Ostrow, 1984; Viney, Benjamin & Preston, 1988). Some suggest that exercise may improve memory, reaction time and cognition by increasing circulation to the brain (Ferrini & Ferrini, 1993). Selecting and participating in exercise programs may also make elders feel better about themselves, resulting in improved intellectual performance and function (Ferrini & Ferrini, 1993).

Lifestyle Choices Dominate

Gerontological research has shown that while one-third of the aging process is due to heredity and biological factors, two-thirds are based on one's lifestyle choices (Kane et al., 1989). As a fitness professional, you cannot stop the aging process, but you can help to minimize the rate at which physical decline occurs by promoting exercise for older adults.

By helping these adults adapt their lifestyle to incorporate healthy exercise habits, you can significantly improve the quality of their life. These improvements may be far-reaching. Participation in a program of regular exercise may produce unexpected mental and emotional benefits for older adults, in addition to desired health or fitness benefits. Studies have shown that people who remain physically and intellectually active maintain their mental alertness and live longer. They also live those extra years in better health than those who simply retreat from engaging in social activities (Spirduso & MacRae, 1990).

THEORIES OF HEALTH-RELATED BEHAVIOR CHANGE

Beginning or modifying an exercise program requires change on the part of your clients, an often difficult task to undertake. The current exerciser may have to increase intensity, duration or frequency, or add another type of exercise to their program to address a new component of fitness. Non-active individuals may have to incorporate a brand new set of activities into their lifestyle, which may require decreasing sedentary pursuits like watching television or reading, and/or setting aside time for exercise despite a schedule filled with active tasks (i.e., volunteer work, caring for friends or family members, or paid work).

To help others make desired behavior changes, you must first understand those factors that encourage or hinder exercise behaviors. Although the field of exercise psychology is relatively new, various health, exercise and psychology researchers already have developed useful theories about how and why people engage in physical activity. Five of these theories will briefly be described, followed by detailed discussions and examples of how to apply behavior-change strategies while working with your own clients. (For more detailed overviews of these and other theories, refer to Willis & Campbell, 1992 or Kaplan, Sallis & Patterson, 1993).

Social Learning/Social Cognitive Theories

These theories emphasize a person's ability to self-regulate their physical-activity behaviors through goal-setting, monitoring progress, and actively working to make social or physical environments conducive to goal attainment (King et al., 1992). Observing others engaging in desired behaviors (such as exercise) and modeling of specific behaviors are important learning tools. Self-efficacy (the belief that one is capable of engaging in a desired behavior) and outcome expectancies (the belief that the behavior will lead to desired outcomes) greatly influence the kinds of new behaviors that are adopted and the degree of effort expended before giving up. A person's self-efficacy can be impacted by personal experience, vicarious experience, verbal persuasion and physiological states (King et al., 1992).

The Health Belief Model

The Health Belief Model (Becker & Maiman, 1975) suggests that the major factors influencing physical activity include perceptions of vulnerability to illness or negative health outcomes, combined with the perception of the seriousness of these outcomes. A person with a strong family history of heart disease, for example, might be highly motivated to improve their cardiovascular fitness as a means of decreasing their chance of having a heart attack. The individual must believe the preventive action (such as regularly running on a treadmill) will help prevent the health problem. Additionally, the perceived benefits of physical activity must outweigh the perceived costs of changing. The person also must have a minimum degree of confidence in their ability to start and maintain the healthy behavior. Lastly, this model suggests the value of using cues as reminders to be active, such as placing jogging shoes by the front door.

The Theory of Planned Behavior

Another influential theory of physical activity is the theory of planned behavior (Ajzen & Madden, 1986), which suggests that the likelihood of successfully performing a behavior is determined by the intent to perform the behavior, and the degree to which we have control over factors related to the behavior. Intentions are affected by our beliefs about the outcomes of behaviors and the value of these outcomes, as well as social influences, such as what we think others want us to do and our degree of concern about conforming to others' expectations. Like the Health Belief Model, the extent to which a person believes in their ability to perform the behavior (to come to the gym and to properly use the weight-training machines, for instance), plays a major role in the intention to even try.

Transtheoretical Model

A relatively recent model that takes into account varying levels of readiness for changing behavior is the Transtheoretical Model (Prochaska & DiClemente, 1982; 1983). According to this model, an individual's readiness to engage in behaviors can be described on a continuum of stages, known as the Stages of Change. Although this theory was originally developed to refer to psychotherapy processes and, later, all health-related behaviors, other researchers have adapted the model specifically to physical activity (Markus, Rakowski & Rossi, 1992). Stages of readiness to be physically active include:

Precontemplation—an absence of serious consideration of changing the behavior (example: "I have never exercised before and I have no desire to start now.")

Contemplation—not engaging in the behavior but seriously considering doing so (example: "I know I should start getting more exercise to help lose weight. Maybe I should join my neighbors on their morning walks.")

Preparation—actually attempting the new behavior or actively preparing to do so (example: asking to join the neighbors' daily walks and buying comfortable walking shoes)

Action—consistently engaging in the behavior at the desired intensity

Maintenance—consistently engaging in the behavior at the desired intensity for at least six months

This model is especially helpful to fitness professionals because it acknowledges individual differences in readiness to exercise at any particular point in time. Markus and Owen (1992) suggest that goals and program strategies must be tailored to the readiness of each individual. It would be inappropriate, for example, to expect a person in the Precontemplation stage to commit to an exercise program. Instead, interventions with a person in this stage would ideally encourage them to consider starting an exercise plan, perhaps by educating them about the benefits of exercise.

In contrast, a person who has been in the Maintenance stage of physical activity for three years apparently has already discovered the benefits of exercise. This exercise "Maintainer" might be quite interested in discussing ways to add excitement to their well-established routine, a topic that clearly would not be appropriate for a person just beginning a physical activity program. Listen for indications of your client's stage of readiness for exercise, and focus on helping them reach the next stage. The ultimate goal is to move them toward the Maintenance stage. Because people can move back and forth between stages, always remain alert for possible changes in your client's stage and adjust interventions accordingly.

It is interesting to note that researchers Barke and Nicholas (1990) specifically studied older adults in terms of these Stages of Change. Although we may be tempted to view older people as set in their ways and unwilling to be active, their sample of 59 adults between ages 59 and 80 scored more highly on

Action, Maintenance and Contemplation of exercise than on Precontemplation. Even among the least active older adults, there were fewer people in the Precontemplator stage than any other stage of readiness. This suggests that even the least active older adults were thinking about engaging in physical activity or were already preparing or attempting to be active. These results suggest that we should recognize the continuing growth potential of older adults, rather than believe stereotypes that imply older adults are unable or unwilling to change.

Relapse Prevention Models

Relapse Prevention Models have identified the factors associated with stopping desired behaviors (Marlatt & Gordon, 1985; 1980; Brownell, Marlatt, Lichtenstein & Wilson, 1986). Initial work focused on why people quit abstaining from undesired behaviors such as cigarette smoking or substance abuse. More recently, the concept of relapse prevention also has been applied to understanding why individuals stop healthy habits. Factors such as negative emotional states, limited coping skills, social pressure to cease desired behaviors, interpersonal conflicts, limited social support, stress and encountering "high-risk" situations can contribute to the cessation of desired behaviors.

When individuals do experience a setback (a temporary lapse from activity), they often believe it will lead to complete failure. Belief in their ability to succeed may be lost after only one slip-up, leaving them feeling out of control, guilty, discouraged and ashamed. This negative thinking can interfere with resuming the desired behaviors (Marlatt & Gordon, 1985). Preparing clients to cope with high-risk situations can prevent relapses. Additionally, helping clients to understand that relapses are

normal, and even likely, can help them cope with setbacks when they do occur, and resume physical activity as soon as possible.

These are just a few of the models that help us to understand the motivators and barriers to physical activity. Generally, models of physical activity take into account some combination of perceived outcomes (including benefits and costs), perceived ability to engage in the physical activity, and positive and negative social influences. What makes these models valuable to fitness professionals is the degree to which they can help promote client success. The next section will address strategies stemming from these and other behavior-change theories, which you can use in your everyday work with all your clients. Descriptions of activity promoting, behavior-change skills and examples of how you might help older clients overcome barriers by using these behavioral skills are included.

Behavioral Change Strategies for Motivating Older Adults to Exercise

Although there are numerous definitions, according to Willis and Campbell (1992), motivation generally refers to factors that initiate behaviors, direct actions and influence when a behavior is discontinued. Often, people talk about motivation as if it were a completely stable, enduring characteristic. Some people just seem motivated to accomplish great things and appear to stay motivated against all odds. How do they do it? In reality, motivation varies over time and according to the task.

Motivation impacts decisions to exercise as well as the likelihood of quitting or maintaining exercise over the long run. It is estimated that approximately half of the people who start exercise programs quit within six months (Willis & Campbell, 1992; Dishman, 1988; Wankel, 1987). Therefore, consistent maintenance of physical activity at the desired level is a major concern. The sad truth is that many clients who seek guidance or leadership with exercise plans will not maintain their programs over the long run.

Although this is by no means an exhaustive list, physical activity/exercise motivators often include health and fitness motives, improving appearance, enjoyment, socialization and psychological benefits (Willis & Campbell, 1992). Some of the factors that influence your clients' motivation to exercise, such as prior experiences with exercise and current fitness levels, are beyond your control. Still, you can impact their motivation in many ways. Physical activity research suggests there are behavior-change strategies that can help people initiate exercise and stay motivated to continue. Sticking to an exercise program typically is referred to as adherence. Sometimes it is discussed in terms of the percent of program goals met (e.g., 70 percent adherence means that 70 percent of the planned exercise was completed). Others simply categorize people as adherent if they meet exercise goals, or non-adherent (a dropout) if they do not meet 100 percent of their program goals.

The behavior-change strategies described below are useful in promoting exercise adherence among all clients. Some, however, may be particularly helpful when working with older adults. As you read the descriptions and examples of these behavior-change strategies, think about your own experiences as a fitness professional, and about times that you did—or could have—employed these strategies with your clients. How would you introduce these behavior-change topics to your clients? What recommendations would you make to those clients based upon these behavior-change principles? Visualizing yourself using these techniques will help you to become comfortable with them and incorporate them into your work.

Setting Exercise Goals with Older Adults

Goal-setting is important for anyone attempting to change behaviors. You can play a pivotal role in teaching clients how to set and evaluate their physical activity goals. It is crucial, however, that your clients' goals be their own. This means that each client should fully agree with the selection of goals and how progress will be measured. Remember that most people quickly lose enthusiasm for meeting others' expectations when those expectations are not compatible with their own motivations and lifestyle. Although terms such as "fitness prescriptions" suggest that an exercise plan can be imposed by an expert upon an accepting client, exercise programs are unlikely to be maintained if the client does not feel they have played a primary role in choosing goals and developing the fitness program.

To illustrate, Mary is a 68-year-old woman who has not engaged in formal exercise for 20 years. She has a busy schedule that includes volunteer work and caring for a seriously ill friend. She makes an appointment with you to discuss using exercise to manage her weight, as well as to improve her energy level and overall health. You may conclude that, ideally, she should be participating in a water aerobics class three times a week, as well as strength training and flexibility exercises at least twice a week. Initially, however, Mary may feel overwhelmed by a program that includes all the physical activities you deem appropriate. The challenge you face is to identify one or two goals that match Mary's current needs and abilities.

The only way to evaluate the fit between your proposed goals and the individual client is to ask each client how they feel about the goals you propose, and how long they think they can continue to meet these goals. Their responses will help you identify the level and types of activity that are appropriate for them. Initial goals may fall far below what you would prescribe for health or fitness benefits, but remember that early success can help your clients gradually work toward more advanced goals. A client may choose to maintain physical activity levels that you deem too low or as neglecting a component of fitness. Do not lose sight, however, of the fact that sustained low or moderate physical activity is infinitely more beneficial than complete withdrawal from activity resulting from feeling pushed into a program that wasn't comfortable.

For Mary, participating in a water aerobics class two times a week may initially be the most challenging goal she feels she can fit into her schedule. In conjunction with this goal, encouraging her to increase lifestyle activity by 15 minutes per day may be appropriate. For example, would Mary be willing and able to climb the stairs to her apartment rather than taking the elevator, or walk down the street to pick up small items at the grocery store? When you meet with her in a week or two to review her progress, she may be willing to consider making time for increased fitness activities such as strength training or flexibility exercises. For now, however, acknowledge the motivation that Mary demonstrated initially and applaud her for setting realistic goals.

The above example illustrates the primary rule of effective goal-setting for fitness professionals: Listen carefully when helping a client set goals, and ensure that the goals are appropriate for their current lifestyle, motivations and stage of readiness for physical activity. This is especially important when working with older adults, who may differ from younger clients in all of

these respects. Taking the time to understand an older adult's concerns, motivation and comfort level with proposed goals enables you to collaborate on setting encouraging and constructive program goals.

An important note about health-fitness/exercise goals: Goal-setting with clients should be contingent upon whether they are seeking health or fitness benefits. While working up to vigorous activity may be desirable for certain fitness gains, moderate physical activity is quite sufficient for attaining health benefits, as indicated in the latest CDC/ACSM guidelines. You will need to educate most older adults (and most clients in general) that the "no pain, no gain" theory is not accurate. Vigorous activity may be necessary for certain fitness gains, but moderate activity can provide substantial health benefits.

The *1996 Surgeon General's Report on Physical Activity and Health* recommends that for health benefits, people of all ages should engage in at least 30 minutes of moderate level physical activity (such as brisk walking) on most, if not all, days of the week. There are several options for attaining the recommended amount of moderate physical activity, ranging from single 30-minute sessions, to breaking up activity into multiple short bouts (of at least eight to 10 minutes each) on a daily basis. Many older adults may come to you seeking health—not fitness—gains. Make your program recommendations appropriate to the type of benefits sought, as well as client interests and lifestyle. Be sensitive to the fact that for some older adults, goal-setting may need to revolve exclusively around increasing lifestyle activity—a very worthy goal in its own right.

The specific steps of goals-setting are described on the following pages. An example of the implementation of each step with an older client is given below each description.

STEPS OF GOAL-SETTING WITH OLDER ADULT CLIENTS

Step 1: Identify the client's primary objective(s).

Ask what they want to accomplish over the long run (months or years) by engaging in an exercise program. They may want to decrease blood pressure, lose weight, improve appearance, perform daily tasks such as carrying groceries or climbing stairs with more ease, decrease stress, meet new people, relieve boredom, improve balance, prevent or manage certain medical problems, improve mood or obtain other positive outcomes. Often, a person's reasons for developing an exercise plan will be discussed at the beginning of your first meeting. In this case, it is appropriate to review their primary long-term objectives when you are ready to develop specific goals.

STEP 1: IDENTIFY THE CLIENT'S PRIMARY OBJECTIVE(S).

FITNESS PROFESSIONAL (FP): Bill, I'd like to be sure I understand what you want to accomplish over the long run so we set goals that meet your needs. Your main reason for beginning exercise is to improve your golf game, right?

BILL: Yes, that's right. I also wouldn't mind being in better shape so I'm not so sore after doing home repair projects.

Step 2: Identify one or two short-term goals that will move your client toward their primary objectives.

Although it is fine to have long-term goals (such as losing 100 pounds or transforming from a sedentary person

to a marathon runner), it is difficult to stay motivated with only long-term goals in mind. Work with your clients to set daily or weekly goals so they can experience smaller, motivating successes on the way to meeting their long-term objective.

Even though the client may want to set multiple goals right away, it is advisable to initially focus on only one or two short-term goals. If necessary, explain to the client that new habits— even healthy ones like exercise—take time to develop. Encourage focusing energy on one or two main goals, allowing clients to succeed in meeting them for a period of time, then add new goals. This is far more productive than having an overly ambitious client try to do too much and then experience the frustration and disappointment of failing.

An important note about selecting short-term goals: It can be very motivating to track and record physical outcomes, such as changes in body measurements. However, try to ensure that your client's short-term goals focus on the process of working toward long-term objectives, rather than solely on outcomes. This is especially important for older adults who may no longer experience rapid physiological improvements. If the primary focus is on the process of completing their exercise routine properly and regularly, clients can feel good about this very important accomplishment, even if they have not seen rapid gains in stamina or strength. Of course, tangible physical or physiological measurements are valuable tools for assessing your client's response to the program and for helping clients improve their health and/or fitness. But for motivation reasons, always have clients set some small, short-term goals focused on personal behaviors under their control (i.e., participating in their walking program or completing their flexibility exercises), rather than outcomes, which can vary widely from one person to the next.

STEP 2. IDENTIFY ONE OR TWO SHORT-TERM GOALS THAT WILL MOVE YOUR CLIENT TOWARD THEIR PRIMARY OBJECTIVES.

FP: It sounds like some exercises to generally improve your flexibility and muscle strength could help you with both your golf game and preparing your muscles for home-repair projects. How would you feel about setting a goal to complete a 45-minute strengthening and flexibility routine in the gym three times a week?

BILL: I think I can do that, as long as you teach me how.

FP: That's what I'm here for. Together, we'll go through each exercise and you can ask me any questions you have. We also will take notes about the exercises that you can keep. That way when I'm not around, you can ask other fitness instructors questions.

Step 3: Once general short-term goals have been agreed upon, define them in **measurable**, **realistic** and **specific** terms.

Goals must be **measurable** so that there is a clear, objective way to determine whether they have been met. Take vague goals and find one or two quantifiable ways to measure progress. For instance, a goal of "working out" is hard to measure, but a goal of completing a pre-planned workout routine in the gym six times over the next two weeks is measurable. It is crucial to have clients track their exercise behaviors, either in a personal notebook or on structured forms.

Goals also must take into account the client's current fitness level, state of readiness to increase physical activity, and lifestyle. Chapter 4 discusses the specifics of pre-exercise screening and fitness assessment in detail. It is imperative that you collect high-quality screening and assessment data from your clients, and use it to determine whether their goals are **realistic**. The trick is to develop short-term goals that are slightly challenging so the person feels a genuine sense of accomplishment when they are met. At the same time, these goals should be designed to produce success and must, therefore, be within the client's ability. Some fitness professionals from Project GRAD, a program to help young adults incorporate physical activity into daily life, employ a helpful "90-percent rule." Under this guideline, a goal is considered realistic only if the client feels at least 90 percent sure they can achieve it. Early successes help to increase client confidence in their ability (both their physical ability and the ability to incorporate the exercise routine into their life), thereby encouraging adherence to exercise programs.

Goals also must be **specific** so plans for meeting them are not left to chance. Vaguely stated intentions such as "mall walking three times this week" are easy to forget or put off (indefinitely). In contrast, people often feel much more committed to meeting specifically defined goals such as "mall walking at XYZ Mall at 8:30 a.m., Monday, Wednesday and Friday, for at least 30 minutes each day." To encourage your clients to think through their plans and increase their commitment, supportively ask them to explain the "what, when, where and how" of meeting their exercise goals.

It also is important that clients explicitly agree to meet their exercise goals. This may take the form of a verbal commitment. Some exercise professionals prefer to put such commitments into writing with a "behavioral contract" that defines physical activity goals and states that the client agrees to make every effort to meet the goals. Written contracts should be signed both by you and the client, and each of you should keep copies for subsequent reference. Such contracts assist in keeping track of client goals, and underscore the importance of their exercise plans.

In addition to specifically defining goals, encourage clients to frequently reward themselves for attaining small goals. "Reinforcement" refers to something that increases the chance that a behavior (in this case, physical activity) will occur again. Your clients can use self-reinforcement to keep their motivation levels high. Perhaps they have wanted to purchase new music, clothing or a piece of equipment for a favorite hobby. If they are able to afford these items and would like to use them as self-rewards, purchasing the item could be made contingent upon meeting their physical activity goals. It often is more practical for clients to reward themselves with favorite activities, such as time spent with a treasured friend, or going to watch the sunset at a scenic spot. The specific types of rewards chosen by different clients will vary greatly; the key is that self-rewards should increase the likelihood that desired physical activity behaviors continue. Other important concepts related to the use of rewards by your clients (and by you as a fitness professional) are discussed later in this chapter.

(After having demonstrated and observed Bill doing each of the recommended exercises, answering his questions and writing each exercise on a workout card for Bill to keep, it is time to specify Bill's short-term goals.)

STEP 3. ONCE GENERAL SHORT-TERM GOALS HAVE BEEN AGREED UPON, DEFINE THEM IN MEASURABLE, REALISTIC AND SPECIFIC TERMS.

FP: Now that we have gone through your exercise routine, let's make concrete plans for the next two weeks. People usually are more successful at sticking to exercise programs when they determine how they will meet their goals. You said you can do the exercise routine you just learned three times a week. What days and times will you come to the gym to do this routine?

BILL: Well, I golf on Mondays, Wednesdays and Fridays, so I don't think those days would

be good. I think I should try coming on Tuesdays, Thursdays and Saturdays.

FP: OK. Is there a particular time you can come on those days?

BILL: I usually feel more energetic in the morning, so I guess morning would be good.

FP: Sounds like a good idea. An exact time doesn't have to be etched in stone, but can you tentatively plan the time you'll come on those mornings?

BILL: Let's say I'll leave my house around 9:00. That will give me time to eat breakfast and read the morning paper.

FP: Great. Even if you end up having to change the time, now you have your exercise session in your schedule. So you will leave for the gym at 9:00 a.m. on Tuesdays, Thursdays and Saturdays, right?

BILL: Yeah, that's what I'll do.

FP: OK. I suggest writing it on your calendar, just like a doctor's appointment or any other important event. When we meet again after your first two weeks, we can discuss how this schedule worked for you.

Step 4: Regularly review successes and problems, revising short-term goals as needed.

This is a critical step that too often is overlooked by clients and fitness professionals. Patterns of exercise successes and difficulties contain a wealth of information that you can use to help your clients. Try to review goals with clients on a weekly or biweekly basis. Congratulate them on all successes, including partially met goals. Too often clients feel like failures when they do not meet 100 percent of their stated goals, and they don't give themselves credit for what was accomplished. You have the opportunity to teach your clients that all effort put toward meeting their long-term objectives and improving their health or fitness is valuable. Remind them to treat themselves to the rewards they have earned if they have not already done so.

Ask successful clients what helped them to succeed. Did they discover especially helpful strategies such as exercising with a friend or attending fitness classes at a certain time of day? Congratulate them on their ingenuity and note the strategies. If your client begins to have difficulties with exercise at a later date, encourage them to employ these strategies again.

Unsuccessful clients can share valuable personal experiences that will enable you to problem-solve with them. In an understanding manner, ask what factors made it difficult for them to meet their goals. Listen for possible patterns. Once you have identified the major problems they encountered, work to generate solutions or modify goals.

Your first concern should be helping the clients feel good about what they accomplished. This will give them the confidence to meet future activity goals. Explain that it is only through trying to meet exercise goals that they can discover which strategies do or do not help them succeed. Explain that instances they see as failures can be helpful if they learn from the experience.

After evaluating successes and problems, clients should commit to a new set of short-term goals. They may opt to keep the same exercise goals, decrease goals that were overly ambitious or challenge themselves with new or intensified goals. In any case, all the previous goal-setting steps still apply. You may make recommendations for revision, but the final selection of the next short-term goals should ultimately rest with the client. As they become regular exercisers, you may formally review goals with them less often (perhaps monthly or every two to three months, depending on the client). Ideally, they will become quite good at tracking their own progress and revising their own goals.

(At second meeting, after Bill has been in his exercise program for two weeks.)

STEP 4: REGULARLY REVIEW SUCCESSES AND PROBLEMS, REVISING SHORT-TERM GOALS AS NEEDED.

FP: Hello, Bill. It's good to see you. How did the first two weeks of your exercise program go?

BILL: I did pretty well the first week. I came to the gym and completed the routine three times, just like we planned. But the second week, I only got to the gym twice.

FP: I want to congratulate you on your successful first week. A lot of people find that beginning a new program is the hardest part. How do you feel about your first week?

BILL: Really good, especially because I had friends in from out of town and didn't get as much sleep as I'm used to.

FP: But you managed to come to the gym and do your routine even though you were tired?

BILL: Yeah.

FP: That's great. What motivated you to exercise even when you were tired?

BILL: I remembered what you said about exercise sessions being just as important as a doctor's appointment—I thought I shouldn't cancel on myself! I guess I didn't want to feel like a quitter, either.

FP: Your exercise time is important and you deserve to take it. I'm glad you decided to keep your appointments during the first week. What made it more difficult during the second week?

BILL: Things just kept getting in the way. I didn't come in on Tuesday because the washing machine broke and my wife wanted me to fix it.

FP: I can see how that might interfere with your plans. Let's think about what you can do when a situation like this comes up again so you'll be able to exercise, but still have time to do the other things you need to do.

BILL: OK. It was kind of an unusual week, but I guess things can always come up at the last minute.

FP: That's right. No matter how much you may want to do your workout, other things are bound to interfere with your plans.

BILL: What do you suggest?

FP: Well, let's look at your experience when the washing machine needed to be fixed. Is there any way you could have taken care of that and still worked out that day?

BILL: I guess I could have done my routine at the gym first, then gone home to fix the washer. It's just that my wife asked me if I could fix it so she could do laundry; I didn't want to make her wait.

FP: And did you mention to her that you had planned to go to the gym that morning?

BILL: No, and I don't think she remembered it, either.

FP: That's not surprising since you recently added this to your schedule. How does she feel about you going to the gym three times a week?

BILL: Oh, she's all for it.

FP: That's great. Do you think she would have understood if you said you'd like to go to the gym before fixing the washer?

BILL: Uh-huh. I guess I just should have reminded her about my plans. She wouldn't have minded waiting.

FP: It's good that she's supportive of your exercise program. Support from family and friends can really help people stick to their regimens. Maybe later we can talk about ways she can help you adhere to your plan. For now, though, what will you do next time something like a household repair comes up before your workout?

BILL: If it's not an emergency, I'll just exercise first.

FP: Good. This experience probably will help you a lot in the future. Now, what goals do you want to set for the next two weeks?

BILL: I'd like to stick with this same routine until I really get the hang of it.

FP: That's a smart idea. I'll note that doing your current routine three times a week is your new goal. Do you want to change the times, or is Tuesday, Thursday and Saturday around 9:00 a.m. still best for you?

BILL: I like that schedule. Let's leave those as the times I'll come.

Summary

Exercise goals that seem simple to you can be intimidating to clients. As the previous examples indicate, discussing and setting specific exercise goals with clients provides a clear plan for building new or modified exercise habits into their lives. Your help in developing these concrete plans can increase a client's confidence in their ability to meet exercise goals. Meeting attainable exercise goals can improve motivation levels and self-confidence, as well. Reviewing client experiences and problems will help you identify issues most likely to encourage or block future success. Lastly, you can teach clients the value of taking pride in their victories, and how to turn their "failures" into learning experiences that will help them reach future exercise goals.

Additional Behavior-change Strategies

In addition to helping older adult clients with effective goal-setting, you can introduce them to a number of other important behavior-change skills that will assist them in meeting exercise goals. You may want to present these concepts to most of your clients, but beware of bombarding them with too many new ideas. Introduce one strategy at a time, and allow clients a few weeks to try it out and discuss their experiences. Introduce new behavior-change skills only as prior skills are mastered or problems are presented suggesting the need to address a different skill area arise. The key is to introduce new ideas at a pace that matches each client's comfort level, interest and abilities.

Because these ideas will be new to many clients, initially you may need to take the role of educator and explain the strategy. However, planning how to implement these strategies should be a joint effort between you and your client. Your initial guidance should prepare your clients to independently use these techniques. When a client is able to tell you that they took the initiative to use one of the strategies on their own, you can enjoy the satisfaction of knowing that you have taught them well.

Using Rewards to Motivate Long-term Adherence

Eventually, your clients may find exercising rewarding in and of itself. Internal rewards, such as improved self-esteem and a sense of personal satisfaction from developing new skills, can be highly motivating (Deci & Ryan, 1985). Note that these motivators reside within clients and their personal perspective; this "intrinsic motivation" to exercise is extremely conducive to long-term maintenance of physical activity or exercise.

Long-term exercisers typically find many inherent aspects of their physical activity give them pleasure and motivate future exercise behaviors (i.e., a sense of accomplishment as they are exercising or post-workout relaxation). Because fitness professionals usually are long-term exercisers themselves, they sometimes expect clients to enjoy the intrinsic rewards of exercise as they do. The reality, however, is that it often takes time to begin enjoying exercise for its inherent internal benefits. Until clients sufficiently develop their physical abilities to focus on pleasurable aspects of their workout rather than how difficult their exertion feels, they cannot be expected to love working out. Even desired outcomes such as improved muscle strength or weight loss cannot be motivators until the person has continued their program long enough to experience these benefits. For some clients, a genuine, internally generated love of exercise may never develop.

Unless clients have begun to report internal rewards, it is crucial to employ external rewards to keep motivation levels high. Such rewards should be planned in conjunction with setting physical activity goals. Clients who do not find exercise to be internally rewarding still can develop and maintain regular exercise routines, but they will need to continue using external rewards.

External rewards for exercise can take many forms. Clients can establish their own reward systems, such as allowing themselves to enjoy a relaxing soak in the spa immediately after they exercise, or treating themselves to a movie each week they meet their exercise goals. You, too, can provide external rewards in the form of praise for achievements or tangible rewards such as prizes for meeting short-term goals. Rewards also can be linked to program monitoring, as in the case of a prominently posted attendance chart documenting each client's attendance, with a gift certificate given for every 10 classes attended.

One word of caution: Remember that the goal is to foster the growth of a client's awareness of internal rewards and intrinsic motivation to exercise. Too much focus on external rewards can foster a reliance upon such rewards (Deci, 1977). To minimize this risk, provide more external rewards when clients are new at exercise behaviors, and gradually decrease them when clients begin to express internal motivation to exercise.

The Social Connection: Using Social Support as Motivation to Exercise

By nature, human beings are social animals. Support from other people is an important tool that may help clients of all ages maintain physical activity. This is especially true of older adults.

As mentioned earlier in this chapter, most older adults are faced with the challenge of coping with multiple losses that often restrict the amount and nature of social contact. Spouses, siblings or treasured friends now may be deceased, while others may have moved away to retirement or assisted-living communities. Physical disabilities or illnesses may prevent friends or other family members from being able to engage in previously enjoyed activities, such as long walks or shopping excursions. Retired individuals who relied upon the work setting as a primary source of social contact may now experience distress over the loss of that environment. Because American society is so mobile, children and other relatives may live in distant cities and be unable to visit regularly.

However, rather than disengaging from society, many older adults desire to rebuild and keep nurturing social connections. If your older clients want to maintain social connections with others and do not already have sufficient opportunities to do so, their physical activity programs can serve a dual function by meeting both exercise and social needs. Exercise programs that take into account the psychological value of social interaction, in addition to the physical benefits of exercise, can become especially prized by older adults.

How can social support be employed to help your clients? It's as simple as teaching them that encouragement will help them comply with their exercise program, and suggesting that they seek support from others on an ongoing basis. Here are some social support strategies to suggest to clients:

✓ Find an enjoyable and reliable exercise partner. If partners aren't readily available in your exercise setting, look to community agencies or programs offered by churches, social groups, university- and community-based senior programs, etc.

✓ Ask friends and family members to be encouraging and positive about your exercise program.

✓ Ask others to remind you about physical activity goals or appointments.

✓ Set up fun "contests" with a friend, and reward yourself based upon meeting an exercise goal, such as attending your chair-based exercise class 10 times without an absence. (Your friend's goal does not have to be exercise-related, although mutual support for exercise would benefit both of you. The main objective is for you to use accountability to someone else as a motivational tool for meeting your exercise goals.)

✓ Add a social element to your exercise program for example, you could arrive at class a little early if it affords the opportunity to chat with other class members.

As a fitness instructor you too can facilitate social support for exercise by fostering social interaction in your programs. Speak with as many of your clients as possible, even if you lead a large class or group. Introduce clients to one another. Incorporate brief exercise activities that require a partner or small groups. Allow clients the space to meet before or after classes to socialize, and encourage participants to plan social events if they desire to do so. Over time, your older clients may develop rewarding friendships with other exercise participants, thereby enhancing their sense of belonging and improving commitment to their program.

It also should be noted that social influences sometimes can make exercise more difficult. A spouse who makes negative comments about an exercise program or friends who always try to persuade your client to go to lunch rather than exercise are good examples. Your client's participation in an exercise program may require adaptation on the part of others, which may or may not be forthcoming.

Although friends and family ultimately may only want the best for your client, they may be experiencing some feelings of neglect or jealousy, or other interpersonal issues that need to be resolved. If you hear a client discussing these kinds of negative influences, work with them to evaluate the impact of such instances on their exercise motivation level. Help clients take greater control over the situation by suggesting that they:

✓ Schedule their contact with unsupportive people *after* they exercise for the day.

✓ Avoid contact with discouraging people altogether.

✓ Try to balance out time with unsupportive people by increasing time with supporters.

✓ Set clear limits for how much time they will spend with unsupportive people.

✓ Mentally prepare themselves to respond to negative comments.

✓ Mentally review why their exercise program is important to them prior to spending time with unsupportive peers.

✓ Explain to an unsupportive person why their exercise is important to them, and ask for the person's encouragement. If the person is willing to try to be more supportive, your client should tell them specifically what they would and would not like them to do. (For example, "It would help me a lot if you wouldn't say, 'Were you off to the gym *again*?' each time I leave the apartment for awhile. But asking how I am progressing in my program every now and then would be nice.")

By helping clients recognize the impact that others' responses may have on their motivation, you prepare them to use positive social support to their advantage, and to decrease the impact of discouraging influences.

Using a Cost-Benefit Analysis to Improve Exercise Adherence

It is basic human nature to want to engage in activities that produce more benefits than costs. Who wants to slave away at a job that offers no pay and no other rewards? The "costs" of physical activity vary from person to person, but could include: the time it takes to exercise, the hassle of getting to the exercise location, muscle soreness, feeling self-conscious about exercising in front of other people, the expense of fitness facility membership or special equipment or clothing, having to miss out on preferred activities, feeling tired after exercise, sweating, etc.

The benefits of physical activity also vary with each individual. Although certain physiological benefits might be expected for most or all people, only the benefits that are personally valued by your clients will motivate them. In this sense, then, benefits are "in the eye of the beholder." If Sally doesn't care about her improved ability to climb stairs without losing her breath, reminding her of this benefit will not be helpful. If Sally values being able to sleep better and having to take less medication to control her high blood pressure, these are more potent motivators to discuss.

Over time, clients' perspectives on the various benefits and costs of exercise will change. They may come to recognize new benefits, and life changes may impact the costs or benefits of certain activities. It is important, therefore, to regularly talk with your clients about the current pros and cons of their exercise program.

Why should we discuss anything negative such as the costs of exercise with clients? To help clients maintain physical activity over the long run, we must be realistic about how they experience that activity. Ignoring the drawbacks of engaging in an exercise program won't make these costs disappear; in fact, unaddressed costs eventually may lead your clients to drop out of their program. By discussing your clients' objections to their exercise routine in an accepting way, you can work with them to decrease or eliminate the costs before they give up on exercise. If a client hates working out alone, perhaps they can find an exercise partner to join them or try some group activities. If feeling tired after exercise is a complaint, perhaps they could schedule exercise sessions in the evening, when feeling relaxed would encourage better sleep.

Discussing costs also lets clients know that their conception of exercise as requiring effort is not abnormal, but a natural part of developing new, healthy exercise habits. This is important, since many sedentary people mistakenly assume that people who exercise regularly are different from themselves—that regular exercisers stick with it because they love every minute of working out. The realization that even physically active people encounter difficulties—but have learned ways to overcome them—will help your clients see that they can learn skills that will help them stay active, too.

As you address client concerns over the costs of exercise, it also is a natural time to review the benefits they reap from being active. Some of these may be immediate, such as feeling more alert or experiencing a boost in self-esteem after an exercise session. Others may be long-term, such as living longer or decreasing the loss of bone density associated with osteoporosis. Help your clients maximize benefits which improves the ratio of benefits to costs. If a client identifies increased energy and weight management as his greatest benefits of exercise, he could consider scheduling his workout in the morning on his busiest days to help him to tackle those days with more energy. Perhaps he'll want to save his occasional high-calorie treats (like dessert) for his exercise days when he burns more calories.

Following is an example of how a fitness professional might help a client improve the ratio of exercise benefits to costs:

FP: Loretta, you mentioned that it's harder for you to stay on the treadmill for 20 minutes because the music in the treadmill room is too loud and you don't like rock 'n' roll. Is that right?

LORETTA: That's right. The blaring music gives me a headache.

FP: So, for you, one cost of exercising is having to deal with loud music you don't like. Can you think of any ways to deal with the situation?

LORETTA: Well, I guess I could complain about the type and volume of the music. Maybe someone would at least turn it down a little.

FP: That sounds like a good idea. Music is supposed to help people work out, not give them headaches, so you have every right to ask that the music be turned down. Rock 'n' roll music may be requested the most so they might not change the type of music, but it wouldn't hurt to ask.

LORETTA: I guess I'll ask them to adjust the volume next time.

FP: I also have another idea. Have you considered wearing radio headphones? You might find that enjoyable since you can play your favorite type of music. You could even wear headphones without playing music to cut down on other noise.

LORETTA: I never thought of that. My grandson wears them all the time, especially on car trips. I wonder if I'd like them....

FP: Maybe you could borrow his to see what they're like.

LORETTA: I'll ask him about it tonight.

FP: Great. The last time we talked you said that one benefit of exercise was feeling pampered because you were taking time just for yourself. Are you still enjoying that?

LORETTA: Oh yes.

FP: I'm glad to hear that. Your exercise time should be a special time just for you.

Directly addressing your client's concerns allows you to help them eliminate or minimize costs. You also can help your client to remember the positive aspects of their exercise program and to increase benefits.

Teaching Clients to Use Reminders to Exercise

"Cues" are simply influences—either planned or coincidental—that remind us to engage in certain kinds of behaviors. Seeing walking shoes by the front door can remind us of our plans to walk that day, or keeping a fitness facility ID card on our key ring can provide ongoing reminders about an exercise commitment. Setting an alarm clock or wrist watch alarm to remind us to leave for an exercise class can be quite helpful.

Unfortunately, some influences also make it harder to engage in exercise. Starting a new book that we don't want to put down can make it difficult to get to a water aerobics class. Having friends drop by unexpectedly to play cards makes it hard to go for a walk. Teach your clients to intentionally use cues to remind them to exercise and, whenever possible, to avoid cues that make it difficult to exercise.

Balancing Convenience and Enjoyment

As mentioned earlier, it is easier to quit an activity that carries more costs than benefits. If an activity is too inconvenient, it will be stopped as soon as the effort outweighs the rewards. Many of us do engage in highly inconvenient activities with some regularity. There are snow skiers, for example, who buy expensive and specialized equipment, drive for hours to reach a ski area, wait in line for lift tickets, brave even the harshest of weather conditions on the slopes, ski to the point of exhaustion, and willingly opt to do it all again as soon as they have another chance. This inconvenient exercise occurs because the people who engage in it experience huge rewards in the form of fun! But if every trip to the fitness facility or every daily walk were as inconvenient as a ski trip, most people simply would not

bother. The difference: People are willing to deal with hassle if an activity is extremely enjoyable or rewarding in other ways.

Therefore, you have two very important lessons to teach clients:

1. **Engage in exercise plans that are convenient.** This applies to a regular exercise routine that can be done even on days when clients have little time or energy for elaborate plans. Going to a nearby fitness facility for a regular class held at a convenient time, or exercising with a videotape at home are good examples of such activities. Hopefully these will be somewhat enjoyable too, but they don't have to be blissfully fun if they are relatively easy to do.

2. **Engage in inconvenient but fun exercise activities, but be realistic about how often they can be done.** For example, one client may love to dress in formal attire and go ballroom dancing, while another likes to drive for an hour to their favorite hiking spot. Clients should be taught to engage in inconvenient but treasured activities when it is realistic to do so, but also to have a set of very convenient exercise options to employ on a daily basis.

Remember enjoyment and convenience when reviewing client progress. Clients who are having trouble meeting exercise goals may need your help to increase convenience. If they hate traffic and driving to the fitness center, perhaps they can carpool with someone. If they dislike early-morning obligations, they should attempt to take fitness classes in the afternoon or evening.

An example of a fitness professional guiding a client through a discussion about balancing convenience and enjoyment follows:

FP: Anna, you say that you are having trouble getting to your stretching class because it is too hard to rush home from your volunteer work, change clothes and get to the class on time. Is that right?

ANNA: Yes. I hate to arrive late, so if I get there and they've already started I just go back home.

FP: I know it's frustrating to join a class in progress, and most people find it hard to exercise when getting to a class becomes a big ordeal. Is there any way we can make your exercise plans more convenient for you?

ANNA: I don't know what to do. I mean, they aren't going to change the class time for me.

FP: Let's consider a few ideas. Some may work and some may not, but at least we can come up with a few possible solutions for you to try.

ANNA: OK. What can I change?

FP: Well, the first thing that comes to my mind is the time you leave your job. Can you leave earlier?

ANNA: I don't know. We set that schedule when I started. I guess it's worth asking to see if I could leave 30 minutes earlier. I wouldn't mind going in earlier to make up the time.

FP: Great. That might be the solution right there, but in case that doesn't work, let's come up with a few more ideas. Is there a way to avoid having to go home to change your clothes before class?

ANNA: I certainly can't work in the clothes I wear for class, and I'd feel silly changing into workout clothes at my volunteer job.

FP: OK. How would you feel about changing clothes here in the locker room?

ANNA: I guess that might be alright. I see other women changing clothes there all the time. I've just never been in the habit of packing up all my things to bring with me.

FP: Well, if you're comfortable with trying it, that may be another solution. You could pack the clothes you'll need for class in the morning, put them in a bag in your car, and then come straight here after work to change clothes. Would that give you enough time to get to class?

ANNA: I think it would.

FP: OK. If these things don't work, maybe we can see if another class starts at a better time for you.

ANNA: Oh, I really like that class. The instructor is great and I like the people in it. I'll see if these other things will work first.

FP: That makes sense. If you really enjoy an exercise class, sometimes it's worth going through a little inconvenience. This week, are you willing to try changing clothes here and

asking your supervisor about leaving your job earlier?

ANNA: I'll do both.

FP: Great. I'll look forward to hearing how things turned out when we meet next week.

As this example illustrates, people often don't consider convenience issues when arranging exercise plans, and may not realize which aspects of the program will be inconvenient until it has begun. Clients may not recognize that it is OK to expect their activity plans to be convenient. They may even chide themselves for not being dedicated enough to their exercise goals when inconvenience gets in the way of goal attainment. You have the opportunity to help them understand the balance between enjoyment and convenience, and to plan their program accordingly.

Teaching Older Adults to Use Self-talk as an Exercise Motivator

Do you ever talk to yourself as you try to complete a difficult task? If so, you aren't alone. All of us have a sort of ongoing internal dialogue within our minds. Sometimes when we concentrate especially hard, we may even "talk through" our thought processes out loud. The statements that we make to ourselves silently (and occasionally out loud) are referred to as "self-talk." So what does this have to do with sticking to an exercise program? A lot.

Self-talk can help us meet exercise goals if it is positive or otherwise motivating. Self-statements such as "I can do it" or "I'll feel much less stiff once I've done my exercises" can help your clients to begin or continue exercising. Self-talk also can be discouraging, as in the case of a person who says to himself, "I don't know why I should bother with all of this work; it's never going to pay off" or "I'll never be able to keep up with the rest of this class." You can help your clients to stay motivated by teaching them how to identify and take control of self-talk related to their exercise goals.

The first step is to identify (to hear) self-talk. This will be easy for some clients; others may find it difficult. Encourage clients to ask themselves what is "going through their minds" when they are feeling discouraged about exercise or having difficulty meeting physical activity goals. This should help them pinpoint the negative thinking that is interfering with their success. They also can learn from positive experiences. Thoughts that help them feel good about exercising can be recalled at times they feel discouraged.

Next, negative self-talk should be corrected. This doesn't require becoming oblivious to reality or trying to think only "happy thoughts." Instead, encourage your clients to try to make their self-talk realistic, rather than unduly harsh, by assessing the accuracy of self-talk. Acknowledging that such statements as "I always mess up" or "I'll never be able to succeed" are exaggerations will help your clients to regain a more realistic perspective.

Sometimes, negative statements will be accurate. (Perhaps your client really *isn't* in the mood to exercise or really *does* find a particular exercise difficult.) In these cases, suggest that they work with you to find solutions, such as determining a way to make their program more appealing or substituting other good exercises for ones that are currently frustrating. While realistic negative thoughts are occurring, however, also ask your clients to try shifting their attention to motivating self-talk. Motivating self-talk often emphasizes the positive effects of exercise: "This will help me to improve my balance" or "I will be so proud of myself when I finish my workout today." Using self-talk to their advantage is a way for your clients to become their own best friends, and

motivate themselves to adhere to their exercise routine.

Helping Clients Plan for the Future: Relapse Prevention Skills

Knowing the factors that contribute to a relapse (ceasing to meet exercise goals) can help individuals predict and plan for future high-risk situations. Factors such as illness or injury, social pressure to not engage in activity, a lack of support for physical activity from friends or family, highly stressful or busy times, and an inability to cope with high-risk situations are just a few of the problems that may hinder progress toward activity goals. Such factors can be difficult for exercisers of all ages.

Fitness professionals should prepare clients to cope with tough situations that are likely to interfere with their exercise programs. Clients must first learn to identify their own high-risk situations. Then they can develop the crucial skills of predicting potential problems and proactively develop plans to deal with them. For example, Mike has difficulty swimming regularly and knows that this will become even harder for him when his family arrives for a three-week visit. He realizes there will be plenty of distractions. Nevertheless, he wants to try to stick with his swimming routine.

A fitness instructor could help Mike turn this challenge into a victory by developing an action plan. Perhaps Mike can re-schedule his swim sessions at the time of day when his grandchildren typically nap, so he won't miss out on time with them. Maybe he could arrange to meet a buddy at the pool at predetermined times, so he will feel obligated to go. Mike is likely to have some good ideas about what will help him to keep swimming. Encourage him to generate his own ideas and to rate their value.

He should try the most highly rated strategies first.

Exercise researchers also have suggested that teaching clients to distinguish between a lapse (a brief period of inactivity) and a relapse (an extended period of inactivity) can be extremely helpful (Dishman, 1991; Marcus & Stanton, 1993). The reason is simple: After missing one or more planned activity sessions, it is common for people to start feeling guilty and ashamed, and to experience decreased self-confidence in their ability to exercise regularly. Additionally, some people will engage in all-or-none thinking, labeling themselves as "quitters" or failures. But if a person has acknowledged in advance that lapses are common, natural and temporary setbacks rather than catastrophic failures, they can more easily forgive themselves and get back on track with their activity plan. Encourage clients to "get back on the horse" as soon as possible after a lapse, even if they must again start slowly. The sooner they resume some sort of physical activity, the better they will feel about themselves, and the easier it will be to get back into their desired exercise routine.

Summary

Each individual will enter your door with a unique mix of personal experiences, motivations, expectations, attitudes and abilities. The specifics of conducting personalized fitness assessment and program design for older adults is covered in detail in subsequent chapters. However, one major theme should already be clear: Teaching and applying the behavior-change strategies introduced in this chapter can facilitate your older clients' progress toward exercise goals.

Using these behavior-change skills is more difficult than merely presenting fitness facts or teaching only the mechanics of fitness training. However, if you strive to use these strategies in your daily work with clients, you are likely to observe positive effects on more than their health or fitness levels. Older clients who frequently face restrictive, negative stereotypes may be grateful for opportunities to use their physical activity program to attain additional social support, increased self-confidence and improved self-esteem, in addition to the physical benefits. When older adults experience growth in their sense of well-being as a result of their physical activity program, remember that it is, in part, a credit to your work.

COMMUNICATION AND LEADERSHIP SKILLS

In both group and individual formats, your leadership skills can significantly affect your older clients' attitudes toward physical activity. First and foremost, it must be clear to all of your clients that you enjoy working with them and are genuinely interested in their well-being. Sincere warmth plus enthusiasm for the exercise skills you are teaching will go a long way toward gaining your clients' trust and increasing their dedication to exercise. However, genuine interest, warmth and enthusiasm are not sufficient in and of themselves. Strong communication and leadership skills also are central to your effectiveness. In their list of optimal leader qualifications, Lewis and Campanelli (1990) concluded that leaders of exercise and health education programs for older adults should be:

✓ trained in the areas of physical activity and aging

✓ able to offer a mixture of fun, purposeful activities

✓ able to relate meaningfully to older adults

✓ willing, interested and empathic

✓ patient with themselves and others

✓ organized in their methods and directions

✓ firm but not authoritarian

✓ trained in group dynamics

✓ trained in CPR and able to recognize signs of overexertion

Fitness instructors should continually strive to improve their professional abilities, just as we expect clients to continue working to improve their fitness levels or general health. As with the behavioral strategies, thinking about how you will apply these communication and leadership skills with clients will help you prepare to use them. After you have read this section, challenge yourself to improve at least one leadership or communication skill. As you make gains in that skill area, try using a new skill. Committing to a process of ongoing professional growth will help you better appreciate a fundamental truth of teaching and leadership: The best instructors learn from their students, even as they are teaching them.

Tips for Communicating with Older Adults

Most of us are familiar with the saying "communication is a two-way street." It is true that the most effective communication requires two willing parties, but the parties must do more than merely speak. They must be able and willing to listen carefully and respond in respectful, constructive ways. Fitness instructors need to be particularly responsive to the communication needs of their older adult clients. Because older adults often are stereotyped or patronized by others, they may be especially appreciative of attentive listening and understanding from their

fitness counselors. The better the communication between you and your clients, the more likely it is that you will hear about problems that could interfere with their program success.

Unfortunately, younger people who have not spent much time around older adults may feel intimidated about communicating with these individuals, and rely upon familiar stereotypes to guide interactions. Hummert, Nussbaum and Wiemann (1992), note that language beliefs and attitudes toward the elderly tend to be negatively biased. These negative stereotypes actually can contribute to instances of communication problems and misunderstandings between generations.

One especially common stereotype is that all older adults have problems communicating based on hearing loss, poor memory or other factors. The reality, though, is that some older clients may have hearing impairments, comprehension problems or difficulties in finding the right words to express themselves, while others may have excellent communication skills (Hummert, Nussbaum & Weimann, 1992).

Younger adults often fail to adjust for individual differences, erring on the side of using what is known as "patronizing speech" or "elderspeak" when addressing older adults (Hummert, Nussbaum & Weimann, 1992). This speech style is characterized by simplification strategies (speaking more slowly, using very simple grammar) and clarification strategies (speaking loudly, articulating very carefully) in addition to basing content upon stereotypes of aging. While adjustments in speech patterns may be well-intentioned, older adults may feel they are being "talked down to."

According to Willis and Campbell (1992), the major keys to effective communication are **attending, listening** and **empathic responding**. These are useful tools for communicating with any clients, but are even more important if clients are different from you. **Attending** refers to focusing your attention on another person rather than on yourself or things going on around you. **Listening** requires actively focusing on both the spoken content and feelings or other messages that are only alluded to.

Empathic responding can be more challenging. Empathy refers to understanding a person's experience from their perspective. Asking yourself, "How would I feel in their situation?" is a good way to understand your client's point of view. Next, your response should accurately acknowledge their experience. Ideally, empathic responses slightly increase the client's awareness of their experiences. Consider the case of Vivian, a 68-year-old client who said to Fitness Instructor Joe, "These weight machines are so complicated. I still get confused about how to use them and have to ask for help, even after three weeks in the program!" Joe simply agreed that some of the machines are complicated and then immediately proceeded with reviewing their proper use. While his technical review may have been helpful to Vivian in some ways, Joe's focus upon only technical issues probably left her feeling somewhat misunderstood and unsupported.

Imagine now that Vivian made the same statements to Fitness Instructor Tim. Before responding, Tim asked himself how he would feel in her situation. Tim decided that he would probably feel embarrassed and/or discouraged. Tim then acknowledged these feelings in the empathic response, "The weight machines can take quite a while to get used to, especially if you haven't used them before. It sounds like you feel badly about having to ask for help after three weeks, but it's great that you ask questions. You are doing a good job of learning the machines—you'll probably find that it will get easier with practice."

Tim's understanding of Vivian's feelings, his reassurance that she was not a failure and praise for asking questions increased her confidence in being able to master the machines. Once she indicated that she was ready, Tim reviewed the use of the problematic machines. This technical review was important to Vivian's safety and success, and it was of even greater value because it followed an empathic response, which motivated her to continue her efforts.

Table 2.1 lists other important communication tips for working with older adults, and their application.

Leadership Skills for Fitness Professionals

Communication with your clients does not occur in a vacuum. It takes place within the context of a relationship in which you hold a special position. You may alternate between acting as a consultant, instructor, counselor, coach, mentor or other roles, depending on the nature of your work and your client's needs. In all of these roles, however, you remain the leader, the person who has primary responsibility for defining how clients can best approach their health and fitness goals.

There are many talents that contribute to a leader's effectiveness. You already may naturally possess many of these abilities, but may need to work on developing some of them. Understanding how groups and individuals may be expected to relate to you over time can be helpful. Skilled fitness instructors also are good at making clients feel emotionally safe, and using feedback for educational and motivational purposes. In addition to these general leadership skills, an appreciation of gender and cultural differences, and creativity in making exercise sessions fun, can encourage clients to get hooked on their exercise program.

Table 2.1

Communication Tips for Working with Older Adults

1. Listen without interruption to your clients' questions and statements before responding.

Instructors often think they must have all of the answers — and FAST — to look competent. But fitness instructors sometimes miss part of what clients are saying because they are busy thinking about how they will answer. To avoid this problem, hear all of what your client has to say before commenting. If needed, remind yourself to take your time and think about what clients say. If you are at a loss for a response, tell your client that you need to think about their question for a moment, then formulate your answer. If you are "stumped," assure them that you will consider their question and get back to them. If you do this, be sure to follow up with an answer as soon as you have researched one.

2. Tune out distractions.

Distractions can occur in the environment (things we see or hear around us), in ourselves (our state of mind or physical condition) or in the speaker (mannerisms or a communication style that make it difficult to pay attention.) Because your clients should be the focus of your attention, eliminate or minimize distractions that make it hard for you to listen. Move to a quiet location if surrounding noise or activity is disruptive. If your mind keeps wandering to a personal issue, silently repeat to yourself everything the speaker says. If the speaker's style makes it hard to listen, respectfully work with the speaker to solve the problem (i.e., ask a soft speaker to speak more loudly).

3. Avoid overuse of filler words.

Sometimes, instructors feel uncomfortable with brief silences and attempt to fill pauses with words. While it often is helpful to acknowledge that you are listening with an occasional "uh-hum," overuse of filler words can become annoying and should be avoided. If you find yourself using too many filler words, take a deep breath and remind yourself that some pauses and brief silences are natural and productive. Smiling and nodding in a supportive manner can show your interest without being disruptive.

4. Avoid patronizing language.

Too often, older adults are spoken to as if they are children, with little regard for their dignity. For example, if a small-framed elderly female fits the "little old lady" stereotype, some adults may unthinkingly address this woman as "dear" or "honey." While the speaker may consider these terms of affection, others may find this approach condescending and offensive. Address older adults as you would any other adults — with respect — in the manner they request. It is not uncommon for older persons to prefer being addressed in a more formal manner (e.g., Mr. Smith, rather than Bill.) If in doubt about addressing an older client by first or last name, ask their preference.

5. Avoid using slang.

Remember that slang often is age-, gender- and/or culturally specific. For instance, it might be appropriate for a 25-year-old woman to use the phrase "you guys" to address her close friends, both male and female. Older women, however, might find such a phrase to be disrespectful. It is best to use mainstream English (or whatever primary language your instruction is in). If you are working with an individual or with group members who are from a similar age group and background as yourself, the use of some slang may be acceptable. Be careful, however, not to patronize clients by attempting to use slang terms you would not otherwise use.

6. Make eye contact.

This demonstrates your interest in each client. A steady gaze can be threatening, but among most American cultures frequently making brief eye contact with clients shows concern and interest. If you are leading a group or class, be sure to make eye contact with each participant.

7. Speak at an appropriate volume and pace.

Nervous and/or enthusiastic leaders tend to speak quite rapidly, often not allowing time for listeners to ask about what was said. If you are a rapid speaker, be conscious of slowing your pace. Additionally, the volume of speech must be loud enough for clients to hear, especially if there is background noise. (Remember that hearing aids amplify all noise — not just your voice — so any background music must be low.)

Ask your clients about volume and pace until you become familiar with their needs. Inquire whether the volume of your voice is OK. Likewise, you can ask clients, "Am I talking too fast?" and adjust accordingly. For hearing-impaired clients, it often is beneficial to slow down the rate of your speech, use some gestures or demonstrations to emphasize points, and look at clients so they can pick up visual cues about what you are saying.

8. Teach new material at an appropriate pace.

It has been noted that although the ability to learn new information remains relatively stable over time, the speed of learning may slow with aging (Spotts & Schewe, 1994). There may be tremendous variation from one client to another, but a good rule of thumb is to allow older adults (and, ideally, all of your clients) to learn at their own pace.

Allow clients to tell you when they are comfortable with what you have taught them and when they are ready to move on. Periodically ask individuals to demonstrate new moves or explain what you have just said. Inquire whether additional practice is desired. If the majority of a class is ready to move on, reassure those who want more practice that you will review the information again, making sure to let them know when. In groups, give clients the option of using a familiar move until they become comfortable with the new one. Provide frequent opportunities for older clients to meet with you or peers to work on new steps or exercises.

9. Visual communication aids should be easy to read.

Older adults' vision will vary widely. To meet the needs of those with vision difficulties, it is best to make writing on chalk boards, signs, flyers and instruction sheets easy to read. Keep visual material uncluttered and brief. Color combinations that give maximum contrast should be used, while varying shades of the same colors (like grays) should be avoided. Pictures or diagrams can enhance some messages, but they should be simple and clear.

Remember that the best way to determine if you are meeting clients' needs is simply to ask. Most clients will appreciate your concern and will attempt to tell you how to help them. An old adage about teaching applies well to fitness instructors working with older adults: It is less important to know all the answers than to ask the right questions.

Each of these skills is important to successful work with older clients, whether in individual or group formats. But there is an almost endless list of other positive leadership characteristics as varied as the number of fitness professionals. Therefore, in addition to developing these skills, recognize your own special strengths as a leader, and use them for the benefit of your clients.

Evolution of Instructor-Client Relationships

Human relationships evolve over time. Understanding the basic stages of relationship development will help you pinpoint and address common client needs, so that your rapport will continue to grow. Table 2.2 summarizes the stages of relationship development, adapted from a group development model by Ward and Preziosi (1994). These same stages also occur within the context of one-on-one work with clients, so they are as relevant to fitness professionals seeing clients individually as they are for leaders of structured exercise classes and facilitators of exercise- related educational programs. Look to your clients' behaviors and concerns for clues about the current stage of your relationship.

Specific tips for instructor behaviors at each stage are given in Table 2.2.

Table 2.2

Stages of Instructor-Client Relationship Development

---

1. Preparation Stage

This refers to fitness instructors' preparation prior to meeting with client(s). Be comfortable with the information to be covered; appearing scattered and disorganized can damage your credibility, while a calm and organized approach can instill confidence.

You will need to:
• Do your homework. Review fitness assessment or exercise tracking information, if applicable. If you are leading group exercise or offering educational programs, be thoroughly familiar with the information you will be teaching.
• Come psychologically prepared (calm, enthusiastic, and focused on the client(s) and your job).
• Finalize content to be covered and presentation methods for structured or semi-structured classes or presentations.

2. Initial Stage

Trust issues are central to your clients, since they are figuring out what your sessions will be like, and how they are expected to behave. In this initial stage older adults in particular may be reluctant to question your authority, to disagree with you or other group members, or to challenge your recommendations. Remember that this is probably not due to unwillingness to cooperate or a lack of interest. For many older adults, you are an expert or authority figure. Initial reluctance to critique your suggestions or to report problems may be based upon long-standing beliefs that one should not question authority. It will take some time and patience to help some of your older clients feel comfortable being candid with you.

You will need to:
• Help clients get acquainted with you (and other group members).
• Set the norm for participation by explaining that client input is respected and essential to success.
• Provide accepting and constructive responses to both positive comments and concerns.
• Point out similarities among your ideas and viewpoints, and those of clients.
• Provide structure and direction.

3. Transition Stage

After you and your clients have worked together for awhile, they may begin to ask more questions or offer challenges. Personal agendas and power issues may surface in groups and classes.

You will need to:
• Continue identifying perspectives and experiences that are shared by you and clients.
• Respond to differences of opinion in a positive manner.
• Keep meetings and classes on track.
• Respond to challenges to your expertise in an open, non-defensive manner.
• With groups or classes, get as many people as possible involved in discussing problems and giving feedback.

4. Working Stage

Relationships are characterized by increased open and supportive communication. In groups or classes, interactions become less instructor-focused, and more exchanges occur between group members. In both group and one-to-one situations, feedback is more readily solicited by clients, and empathy among clients and fitness instructors often is high.

One danger that may arise during this stage is that clients' or instructors' desires for approval or acceptance may take priority over exercise goals. For instance, Richard states that he has missed the last three power-walking classes because he has been busy planning a social event for his condo community. In an attempt to maintain a warm and positive relationship with Richard, his fitness instructor may refrain from reminding Richard that walking remains vitally important to his health and well-being, even when he is busy. Similarly, clients who have bonded well with their fitness professional may be reluctant to report when strategies proposed by the instructor are not working well for them.

You will need to:

• Encourage members to honestly report what does and doesn't work for them on a continual basis.
• Encourage clients to turn ideas into action.
• Remember that your primary role is to provide expert guidance. Tactfulness always is required, but don't hesitate to gently challenge clients or constructively critique their performance when needed. Your main role is not to be a friend, but rather a coach.
• Interpret individual or group behavior when it will help clients. (Example: "I notice that fewer people are coming to class during this holiday season. I know this is a very busy time for some of you, but making time for exercise can help you to stay healthy and reduce tension if you have a lot of holiday stress to deal with. Congratulations for being here today! Please encourage your friends to keep coming, too!")

5. Final Stage

This is the time to terminate work with an individual or group. Emphasize what your clients have accomplished, and challenge them to carry on with skills they have learned. This also is the time for the fitness instructor to summarize what has been learned and to establish a sense of pride and closure. Many clients naturally will begin to emotionally distance themselves; increased absences for individual sessions or groups is not uncommon.

You will need to:
• Address any remaining questions or concerns.
• Acknowledge the ending of the current relationship and emotions related to the change (e.g., apprehension, sadness, etc.).
• Summarize the accomplishments of individual clients, classes or exercise groups.
• Reinforce your clients' exercise-related changes and insights.
• Ensure that your clients know how to get more information and support, as needed.
• Ensure that clients have the knowledge to maintain healthy physical activity behavior changes.
• Confirm each client's future exercise commitment(s).

6. Evaluation Stage

Focus on assessing your performance as a fitness instructor and your clients' experiences working with you or attending your class or group.

You will need to:
• Follow up with your clients regarding their experiences and suggestions, in person and/or through evaluation surveys.

Use this information to improve your skills as a fitness instructor. An isolated comment might be coincidental, but the validity of suggestions or criticisms that come from two or three people always should be seriously considered. When appropriate to do so, modify your behaviors and programs to address these issues.

As this discussion has indicated, your work with older adults will not be limited to conveying information. These relationships will grow and change over time, and the stage of your relationship may influence the kind of information you choose to share or how you communicate it. This insight and flexibility can help you nurture the development of your working relationships.

Instructor Responsibilities During Individual and Group Sessions

Just as relationships with individuals and groups grow over time, there is a natural progression of events that should occur each time you meet with clients or lead classes. It is your responsibility to smoothly guide clients through each of these steps, making your time with them productive and focused. For the sake of efficiency, the term "session" will refer to both individual work and group activities.

Step 1: Beginning the session. Introduce yourself and let clients know that it is time to begin. Explain what you will be doing that day and how you expect them to participate. This is especially important when working with new clients or class members. Reassure clients that they can participate at their own pace, and they will not be expected to engage in movements that they are unable to perform or are uncomfortable doing.

Concentrate on:

✓ setting a positive tone (*I'm glad to see each of you here today!*)

✓ focusing clients' attention on exercise (*Now it's time to get our workout going.*)

✓ explaining what to expect (*Today we'll talk about how your routine is going, and I'll teach you a new exercise for your hamstrings.*)

✓ reviewing prior performance, if applicable (*Last class we learned a new move and all of you started to get it. Is everyone comfortable with that move?*)

Step 2: Leading the session. This is the body of your session, when the bulk of the exercise, education and/or discussion will occur. (* indicates leader behaviors that are especially important for older adults.)

Concentrate on:

✓ providing clear instructions (*First let's review your exercise chart. How many times did you swim last week?*)

✓ allowing adequate time for questions* (*Do you have any questions about where you should feel this stretch?*)

✓ presenting options for modifying types of movements, intensity, etc.* (*If you aren't comfortable with this new move, you can march in place, like this [demonstrating].*)

✓ giving plenty of genuine, positive feedback (*You are showing some great endurance.*)

✓ actively engaging clients' participation (*Who can tell me the purpose of this exercise?*)

Step 3: Closing the session. This sets the tone for the feelings clients carry away from the session, so be sure to close on a positive note! Review what has been accomplished and what clients should be doing until you meet again.

Concentrate on:

✓ summarizing your clients' achievements (*Everyone's form looked terrific today.*)

✓ restating clients' "homework," if applicable (*So this week you'll buy a new pair of aerobics shoes and will walk three times.)*

✓ expressing the expectation of seeing them again *(I'll look forward to our next appointment on Thursday morning.)*

By carefully performing each of your duties as a fitness leader, you will confirm that you are well-prepared and that your clients' time with you is well spent.

Creating a Safe Environment for Older Adults

To facilitate the success of your older clients in meeting exercise goals, you must create a safe environment for them. We commonly think of safety for exercise program participants in terms of physical safety issues (Is the floor dry and the surface smooth? Are participants properly warmed up before doing strenuous exercises?) These are extremely important issues for all clients, especially since injury or illness is seen as a barrier to regular exercise by 19 percent of men and 34 percent of women older than 65, as opposed to only 8 percent of men and 9 percent of women aged 25 to 44 (Stephens & Craig, 1990). In a review of the challenges of physical education of older adults, Cousins and Burgess (1992) reported that chronic conditions may indeed put some older adults at increased risk of aggravation or pain, or require physical activity modifications. Research has suggested, however, that older adults generally are not more injury prone than younger adults (Clarkson & Dedrick, 1988), although fears of injury increase significantly with age (Stephens & Craig, 1990).

Then why might even healthy older adults at low risk for injury be overly fearful of exercise? The answer rests in a frequently overlooked aspect of client safety: the concern for psychological safety. Perceived risk of injury or bad health outcomes is subjective. As a result, you may feel that some clients' concerns about injury are realistic, while other clients allow an exaggerated fear of injury to unnecessarily prevent them from exercising. Most older clients will not engage in physical activities they perceive as dangerous, no matter how adamantly you insist that they should.

Increased psychological comfort with exercise programs can dramatically improve program adherence. Help older adults safely exercise at or near their physical ability by accurately identifying and minimizing both physical and psychological risks of exercise. Subsequent chapters suggest specific components of program design intended to minimize the risk of physical injury to your older clients. Table 2.3 presents a few common psychological risks of exercise for older adults, some of which are based upon the work of Cousins and Burgess (1992), and others that are based upon fitness professionals' experiences. Suggested strategies for helping older clients to overcome each of these risks are given in Table 2.3.

Types and Uses of Feedback to Clients

A primary task shared by fitness instructors is to provide clients with helpful feedback. Different types of feedback serve different functions. Feedback may be technical, as when you comment on a client's form as they use a piece of equipment or perform an exercise. It also may take the form of counseling, as when you work with clients to set new physical activity goals or problem-solve their barriers to exercise. Another intent of feedback may be to reassure clients about their performance, or to enhance their motivation.

Positive feedback is a response that tells a person or group what they are doing right (Hughes, Ginnet & Curphy, 1993). Telling an exercise class "I see that everyone is moving their weights

Table 2.3

Common Psychological Risks of Exercise for Older Adults

1. Risk of Embarrassment or Ridicule. This risk may be especially serious for older adults who never have been physically active or who are attempting to engage in exercise after an extended break. All clients may be susceptible to the risk of embarrassment, but remember that older adults are attempting to engage in an exercise plan despite societal messages that exercise is only appropriate for younger adults, that older adults are too frail for exercise, or too old to develop new skills. (Hence the term, "You can't teach an old dog new tricks.") It is no wonder that some older adults fear criticism.

To Help Your Older Clients: Acknowledge your client's wisdom and courage in committing to their health or physical fitness by exercising. Reassure them that the vast majority of individuals in exercise programs are preoccupied with their own performance, leaving little time to worry about what others are doing. Predictions of failure from family members or others, if they occur, can be used as a motivator to succeed and to prove skeptics wrong.

2. Risk of Facing Diminished Physical Abilities. This problem can be especially difficult for former athletes or former regular exercisers who have not been active in a long time. Many older adults may compare their current performance to what they could do when they were younger, and finding out that they can do less than expected can be a demotivating blow to self-esteem. Older clients who note declines in their abilities may be reluctant to continue exercise activities that painfully remind them of these changes.

To Help Your Older Clients: Encourage them to measure progress from their present starting point. We would never expect a person of any age who has not exercised for a while to be able to automatically perform as they did when they were exercising regularly. Additionally, remind clients that individuals of any age have plenty of room for substantial gains in physical abilities. Even if their current performance feels disappointing, with time and consistent participation in their exercise routine, they may be pleasantly surprised at how much they can improve.

3. Risk of Confronting Ageist Stereotypes of Physical Beauty. Given society's obsession with youth, older women may feel acutely self-conscious while exercising, particularly if the setting is a facility where slim, well-toned young women work out. Males, too, can suffer from damaged self-esteem when comparing their own physiques to those of well-conditioned young men who exercise at the same facility.

To Help Your Older Clients: Remind them that the only people they need to please are themselves. Suggest they concentrate on the benefits from participating in an exercise program regardless of how they fit into the visual profile of others attending a facility. Point out, too, that by actively taking steps to improve their health, appearance and self-esteem by exercising, they are improving to their own physical attractiveness.

These are just a few of a wide variety of psychological risks your clients may associate with physical activity programs. By supportively encouraging them to come to terms with these and other risks, you will free your clients of restrictive barriers to exercise and fears that may impact many aspects of their lives.

slowly and with control; that's great!" is an example of positive feedback. In contrast, **negative feedback** is a response that tells a person or group what they are doing wrong (Hughes, Ginnet & Curphy, 1993). For example, "I see some people getting into the pool to swim laps without doing any initial stretching or warm-up. That's not good for your body, which needs time to prepare for exercise." Negative feedback is necessary to teach clients to avoid errors that could put them at risk for injury.

It is not helpful for clients to hear that they are doing something wrong if they are not informed about how to correct the problem. Therefore, negative feedback should be immediately followed by corrective information. **Corrective feedback** is a response to observed behavior that provides specific instruction on how to improve the technique or performance. Even if clients are not in danger of injuring themselves, corrective feedback that can lead to improved health or fitness benefits should be given. This type of feedback also can be used to correct client misconceptions about their exercise program, the use of behavior-change skills or fitness in general. In the case of teaching physical movements, it often is helpful to supplement corrective feedback with modeling (demonstrating) the proper form.

Prevent clients from jumping to the conclusion that they are doing everything wrong by giving negative and corrective feedback in conjunction with positive feedback. Researchers and leadership specialists have suggested the "sandwich technique," which simply refers to placing negative and corrective feedback between two instances of positive feedback (Hughes, Ginnet & Curphy, 1993). When commenting on client performance, start on a positive note and end on a positive note. For example: "Frank, you are doing a great job of keeping your back against the mat as you start your sit-ups. Try not to pull your head forward; that puts strain on your neck. Keep your neck and elbows back like this (while demonstrating proper form). Your form on your floor exercises is really improving."

Remember to give positive feedback as soon as clients improve their form or correct mistakes. Don't wait to give encouragement until they have perfect form because it may take many attempts for them to succeed. To keep clients motivated, give positive feedback about each successive step toward the desired outcome, in conjunction with corrective instructions. (Example: "That is much better, Frank! Now see if you can lean your head back even farther. Good work.")

Redirective feedback attempts to switch the subject under discussion by keeping conversations on target. For example, a personal trainer might have to change the subject from a client's extended discussion of his vacation to strength-training goals. Redirection can also be used to alter the way a process is being handled. For instance, if an experienced aerobic dance participant is commenting on a new class member's performance in a hurtful way, the instructor could use redirection to guide how feedback should be given. The instructor might say, "Rose, I'm sure you remember how hard it was trying to learn the steps we use in our classes. It seems like an awful lot to remember at once. Would you be willing to demonstrate just one of the steps?" Redirection can be relatively painless for the redirected clients if it is done with respect and sensitivity.

Keep in mind the tasks to be accomplished during your meetings with individual clients or in groups or classes. Discussions that trail into extended tangents quickly get boring or seem chaotic, leaving clients questioning the value of participating. Therefore, try to stay on track with what you planned to accomplish, using redirection when needed.

This does not mean, however, that fitness professionals should become tyrants, never tolerating the slightest bit of non-exercise commentary. Some older adults are deprived of adequate social contact, or may want to use their exercise program for social connection, as well as health benefits. They may want to share information about themselves to help you and others get to know them, and may ask you details about yourself and your life.

Other older clients may feel a natural and compelling need to make sense of new information by relating it to their past experiences. In such cases, older clients need room to share information that may not be directly related to their health or fitness programs. Accept and welcome this type of communication if it helps your clients to bond with you or others in a fitness program, or to generally feel understood and cared about. Think of redirection as a tool to help you maintain a comfortable balance between accomplishing exercise-related tasks and your clients' needs for individual expression.

If you find yourself using redirection techniques often, try to examine why. The need for frequent redirection might be expected if you are dealing with older adults who suffer from cognitive impairments that lead to disorientation, short-term memory problems or difficulty paying attention. But with clients without cognitive difficulties, the need for frequent redirection might signal problems with the information you are presenting. Is the material interesting to your clients? Is it clearly relevant to their lives? Distractions also can make it harder for clients to stay on task; is there activity or noise in the background that makes it hard for clients to focus, or hear what you are saying? Are your questions and instructions clear so clients understand the desired response? A client's response may seem off-target simply because they don't understand what kind of response you want. Lastly, difficulties staying on track almost always suggest a client's need for more consistent positive feedback when they are on track.

No matter what type of feedback you are giving, following certain rules will increase the chance that it will be beneficial. Hughes and colleagues (1993) suggest a number of tips for improving feedback skills. Among others, they suggest that feedback should always:

✓ Be helpful. (Emphasize behaviors that are under the client's control.)

✓ Be specific. (Give a clear understanding of what behaviors need to be changed and how to change them.)

✓ Be timely. (Give feedback as soon as possible after the behavior is observed.)

If the immediate situation is not a good time for your client to hear

feedback (for example, they are surrounded by people and you know that they would be embarrassed by receiving corrective feedback in front of others), offer the feedback at the earliest appropriate opportunity.

✓ Include positive and corrective feedback. A mix of recognition for what is right, plus ongoing suggestions for improvement, can optimize your clients' ability to develop the skills you are teaching.

A final note: Feedback may elicit different feelings in different listeners. Something that you said for the sake of simple redirection may be interpreted as negative by one client and positive by another. Remember that the overall goal of feedback is to help your clients. Carefully observe the effects of your feedback on each person. Over time, you will learn how particular clients receive your comments, allowing you to tailor your feedback so that it has the intended effect.

Sensitivity to Gender and Ethnic/Cultural Differences

At first glance, the differences between a fitness professional and their client may seem to far outweigh the similarities. Fitness instructors are called upon to work with clients from different age groups, genders, ethnicities, cultures, economic situations, life experiences, personalities, etc. Don't become overwhelmed by the diversity; successful fitness instructors approach differences as interesting aspects of clients that deserve both consideration and appreciation. Each client's beliefs, perspectives and lifestyle will impact their health and fitness goals and the ways in which they will want to meet them. Exercise programs must take into account the individuals for whom they are designed, and must work with that person's values. Appreciating differences will help you consistently demonstrate respect and acceptance. Always remember that if all clients were clones, your job would be pretty dull!

Clients' exercise interests may be highly influenced by cultural messages about appropriate male and female behavior. Much of older adults' life experiences occurred during times that were more restrictive in terms of gender-appropriate behavior. Although most older clients may have revised their perspectives many times over the years, and some may always have been progressive in their thinking about sex roles, many older adults may be influenced by historic notions of "acceptable" male and female behavior. For example, some older females may be concerned with issues of modesty, finding the scanty workout clothes worn by some people at a fitness facility offensive. A few older male and female clients may feel strongly that women have no business in the weight room. Older males may think participating in aerobic dance, yoga or flexibility classes is not masculine. Older women and men may prefer exercise groups of the same gender over co-educational instruction.

As a fitness professional, your main task is to help your clients engage in exercise activities that best serve their health and fitness needs and interests. As much as possible, recommend activities that are a good match for client perspectives, as well as the desired outcomes. That is not to say that you should never challenge a client to broaden their thinking. It may be extremely helpful for an older woman who is experiencing difficulty with daily household tasks that require upper body strength to try some strength exercises using weight-training equipment. Similarly, an older man who attends a stretching class might benefit from increases in flexibility and be pleasantly surprised to see other males in the room.

Remember to be sensitive to clients' feelings. Provide gentle encouragement and occasional challenges to clients' thinking without attacking entire perspectives. As your relationship develops and you patiently encourage new activities, your older clients may become willing to branch out into some new exercise behaviors. If this does not happen, continue working within the parameters of their current attitudes to meet the primary objective of keeping them actively engaged in their exercise program.

Cultural and ethnic differences also can impact your work. In a discussion on communicating with older adults of different ethnic and cultural backgrounds, Joan Wood (1989) noted that most research and health-related programs have been developed from white, urban, middle-class models that ignore variations. She notes that health professionals are more likely to come from upper-class non-minority backgrounds, and that there is a great need to develop effective cross-cultural communication skills to better serve all older adults. Some important points from her discussion and suggestions for improving cross-cultural communication skills follow.

Culture refers to socially transmitted beliefs, institutions and norms for behavior, while ethnicity refers to a shared history, culture and sense of peoplehood. Culture and ethnicity are inseparable from other components of an individual's identity. Lifelong patterns of socialization within an ethnic group play a major role in shaping personality, so sensitivity to culture is crucial to individualizing the services you provide to older adults.

One example of how ethnic differences may impact your work is the variation in the social status of older adults in many minority cultures vs. white, middle- and upper-class American cultures. Although older adults from minority groups may be isolated or segregated from the mainstream white culture, remember that they may be fully integrated within their own cultural group. Unlike white older adults, who often experience decreases in respect and power with age, older adults from some ethnic minority groups occupy positions of great honor, respect and authority. In some minority cultures, older adults frequently provide a home for younger children and grandchildren, use their own homes as the gathering place for culturally important events, and preside over important community and family decision-making processes. In economically disadvantaged situations, older adults may provide the most stable income (from retirement or benefits programs) and take on substantial parenting responsibilities for grandchildren whose parents work.

While the roles of older adults vary dramatically even among the same culture, this example highlights several important implications. First, failure to treat older adults with sufficient respect may impair your ability to build a trusting and positive relationship with them. The best approach is to consistently show in your actions and words that they are valued. This will increase the likelihood that your client will share important information with you and continue to invest in working with you to meet their health or fitness goals.

It can be dangerous to make generalizations about clients' lifestyles. For instance, you cannot assume that all retired men sit home most of the day, and have no obligations other than addressing their physical activity goals. Take the case of an African-American older adult who holds a position of authority in his church, does extensive volunteer work with agencies in his community, and frequently chairs committees that organize and implement important cultural events. This client may be too busy for an exercise program that demands two hours in the fitness facility four times a week. Inquire

about the lifestyle of each client, rather than make assumptions about what the client should be willing and able to do.

Here are some suggestions to increase sensitivity to the needs of older adult clients from varied cultures:

✓ Treat all older adults with respect. Do not minimize the importance of their other activities, and do not patronize them.

✓ Understand that cultural beliefs may have a large impact on ideas about health and fitness. Some cultural beliefs actually may suggest that physical activity is an undesirable or unattractive behavior, or that health outcomes are mostly determined by factors other than personal exercise habits (such as spiritual or religious forces, or emotional states). Beliefs about exercise or physical activity will influence clients' compliance with their exercise programs, as well as their motivation. As you develop program goals and assess progress, strive to understand the beliefs that may be influencing your client. You don't have to agree with all of their beliefs, but show respect for them, and make exercise recommendations that fit their belief system.

✓ Seek out expertise when needed. Read about or attend training on cross-cultural communication. Enlist the help of cultural mediators from various ethnic groups, either on a formal basis (working with ethnic minority staff) or informal basis (receiving advice from friends, co-workers or other members of ethnic groups).

✓ Be empathetic. As much as possible, listen to your client's experience and attempt to see their perspective. Preferring our own way is not the only barrier to empathy. Automatic assumptions that clients' values, viewpoints and reactions will be the same as ours also should be avoided.

Currently, minority elderly populations are growing more rapidly than the white elderly population. Life expectancy for non-whites born in 1985 is 68 years, compared to 74 years for whites. However, the life expectancy of minority group members is gradually increasing. In 1980, 12 percent of the population older than 65 was non-white. It is estimated that by 2050, 18 percent of the 65-and-older population will be non-white (Lesnoff-Caravaglia, 1987). This implies that the already vital need for exercise programs designed and offered to minority elders will only increase.

Working with clients who are different from you need not be intimidating. It can be one of the most enjoyable and exciting challenges of your work as a fitness professional. If you approach all of your clients with respect and a willingness to learn about their perspectives, your working relationships will be productive and rewarding.

The Fun Factor: Leader Strategies for Making Exercise Enjoyable for Older Adults

Appreciating and using humor is one way to make work with older clients more fun. You also can keep classes interesting with enjoyable music. Periodically introduce new concepts, exercises or movements to keep both individual and group programs stimulating. Brief descriptions of some of these strategies follow, but there are many more possibilities. Combine your own creative energy and knowledge of your older adult clients to build more enjoyment into your exercise programs.

Humor

You can take your work seriously without always taking yourself seriously.

Human resource research has determined that leaders who use humor often are perceived as both more likable and effective. Environments where humor is welcome result in benefits that range from increased motivation, creativity, satisfaction and productivity to decreased stress. Humor is a wonderful tool for capturing your clients' attention and having fun as you lead exercise classes or work individually. According to Dean (1993), humor:

✓ shows people that you are approachable and "down to earth"

✓ conveys confidence in your relationship with clients

✓ decreases tension or anxiety if clients are nervous

✓ puts issues into perspective in a non-threatening way

✓ demonstrates that you value and encourage spontaneity

Here are a few tips for appropriate uses of humor, adapted from the work of Ozzie Dean (1993):

1. Making fun of yourself from time to time is OK, but do not make fun of others.

2. Laugh with others, not at them. Don't tell a funny story about someone in the group or known to the group, unless you have first obtained their permission to do so.

3. Avoid any sort of age-related, ethnic, sexist or other type of put downs.

4. Show clients that it is OK to laugh. If you are able to relax and laugh from time to time, you have given them permission to do so, too.

Try to be open to using humor to make the exercise skills you are teaching or the activity you are leading more interesting. Humor should not detract from your exercise goals for the group or person, but should contribute to clients' motivation.

Music

Although there may be tremendous variation, appropriate use of music can greatly enhance exercise experiences, especially in structured exercise classes. Frequently, Big Band music, show tunes or instrumental music is enjoyable to the greatest proportion of older clients. However, avoid making assumptions about the types of music that older adults should or will like. The best way to learn about their music preferences is to ask; you may even want to request specific suggestions.

No matter what the type of music, volume should be kept low. High volume may interfere with an older client's ability to hear your instructions and can be especially problematic if they wear a hearing aid. The rhythm should be easy to follow and the tempo appropriate for clients' physical abilities and skill levels. By listening to older adults' input, you can determine the degree to which music can enhance their exercise activities.

Other Ways to Add Novelty and Variety

People naturally enjoy activities that are interesting and fresh, which usually requires adding variety, such as occasional changes in exercise routines. Remember that some older adults may require more time to learn new movements or skills. Experts in programming for older adults frequently warn fitness instructors to avoid overwhelming older clients with too many sudden changes to established routines.

Whether you are leading fitness classes or working with clients on a one-to-one basis, the rate of change should be emotionally and physically safe, and comfortable for the client. New steps or equipment should be introduced gradually, with plenty of time for practice. Remember that successful experiences are good motivators, whereas feeling lost or unable to perform new movements can be embarrassing and frustrating. Ensure success with new movements by keeping them simple. In the case of fitness classes, offer frequent demonstrations of movements for different ability levels and encourage modification of movements as needed. Frequently returning to familiar basic movements such as marching in place will enable even new participants to experience success often. When working with older clients, provide lots of positive feedback as they try new exercises or activities and make sure that plenty of time is spent on tasks they perform well.

Tips for Handling Nervousness or Anxiety

No matter how knowledgeable you are about providing fitness instruction, leading new kinds of classes or working with new kinds of clients can sometimes make even seasoned fitness professionals nervous. If you do find yourself feeling anxious, the following tips may help.

Before the session:

✓ Be sure you're at ease with the material by rehearsing your role.

✓ Visualize yourself as a confident and successful fitness instructor. Picture the best-case scenario of how you'd like your appointment or class to go.

✓ If needed, enlist the help of an experienced co-leader the first few times you do a new type of workout.

During the session:

✓ Focus on the value of what you are teaching, and how it will help your clients. (This takes your focus off yourself and places it back on your clients.)

✓ Practice empathy. Focusing on your clients' perspectives not only helps you to serve them better, but also takes attention away from your own anxiety.

Conclusion

An older client's exercise-program satisfaction and participation is often directly related to their relationship with you. Your knowledge and application of behavior-change principles can help clients develop and sustain new exercise habits. Showing interest and frequently giving sincere praise are especially motivating to older adults, who can be deprived of sufficient positive contact. Because they may not have recent exercise experiences or physically active peers to help them understand what to expect, your support becomes even more important when older adults are just beginning to exercise.

Invest time and energy into getting to know your clients. Nurture your relationships with them by showing acceptance and interest in their well-being. Make an ongoing effort to improve your own communication and leadership skills. In addition to enhancing your own professional abilities, the uplifting effect you will have on many of your older adult clients may become its own reward.

References

Ajzen, I. & Madden, T.J. (1986). Prediction of goal-directed behavior: Attitudes, intention and perceived behavioral control. *Journal of Experimental Social Psychology,* 22, 453-474.

Barke, C.R. & Nicholas, D.R. (1990). Physical activity in older adults: The stages of change. *Journal of Applied Gerontology,* 9, 2, 216-223.

Becker, M.H. & Maiman, B.A. (1975). Sociobehavioral determinants of compliance with health and medical care recommendations. *Medical Care,* 13, 1, 10-24.

Brown, D.R. (1992). Physical activity, aging, and psychological well-being: An overview of the research. *Canadian Journal of Sports Science,* 17, 3, 185-193.

Brown, D.R. (1990). Exercise fitness and mental health. In C. Bouchard, R.J. Shephard, T. Stephens, J.R. Sutton & B.D. McPherson (Eds.) *Exercise, Fitness and Health: A Consensus of Current Knowledge* (607-626). Champaign, Ill.: Human Kinetics.

Brownell, K.D., Marlatt, G.A., Lichtenstein, E. & Wilson, G.T. (1986). Understanding and preventing relapse. *American Psychologist,* 41, 765-782.

Burlew, L.D., Jones, J. & Emerson, P. (1991). Exercise and the elderly: A group counseling approach. *Journal for Specialists in Group Work,* 16, 3, 152-158.

Cantor, M. (1991). Family and community: Changing roles in an aging society. *The Gerontologist,* 31, 3, 337-346.

Carstensen, L. & Turk-Charles, S. (1994). The salience of emotion across the adult life span. *Psychology and Aging,* 9, 2, 259-264.

Clarkson, P.M. & Dedrick, M.E. (1988). Exercise induced muscle damage, repair and adaptation in old and young subjects. *Journal of Gerontology: Medical Sciences,* 43, 4, M91-96.

Cousins, S.O. & Burgess, A. (1992). Perspectives on older adults in physical activity and sports. (Special Issue: Educational Gerontology in Canada). *Educational Gerontology,* 18, 5, 164-481.

Davis, K. (1986). Paying the healthcare bills of an aging population. In A. Pifer & L. Bronte, (Eds.) *Our Aging Society: Paradox and Promise.* New York: W.W. Norton & Co.

Dean, O. (1993). The effective use of humor in human resource development. From J.W. Pfeiffer (Ed.) *The 1993 Annual Developing Human Resources,* San Diego, Calif.: Pfeiffer and Company.

Deci, E.L. (1977). Intrinsic motivation: Theory and application. In D.M. Landers & R.W. Christina (Eds.) *Psychology of Motor Behavior and Sport,* (388-396). Champaign Ill.: Human Kinetics.

Deci, E.L. & Ryan, R.M. (1985). The general causality orientations scale: Self-determination in personality. *Journal of Research in Personality,* 19, 109-134.

Dishman, R. K. (1991). Increasing and maintaining exercise and physical activity. *Behavior Therapy,* 22, 345-378.

Dishman, R. K. (1988). Overview (1-9). In R.K. Dishman (Ed.) *Exercise Adherence: Its Impact on Public Health.* Champaign, Ill.: Human Kinetics.

Ferrini, A.F., & Ferrini, R.L. (1993). *Health in the Later Years.* (2nd ed.) Dubuque, Iowa: William C. Brown.

Himes, C. (1992). Social demography of contemporary families and aging. *Generations,* XVII, 3, 13-16.

Hughes, R.L., Ginnet, R.C. & Curphy, G. J. (1993). *Leadership: Enhancing the Lessons of Experience.* Homewood, Ill.: Irwin.

Hummert, M.L., Nussbaum, J.F., & Wiemann, J.M. (1992). Communication and the elderly: Cognition, language, and relationships. (Special Issue: Communication and aging: Cognition, language, and relationships). *Communication Research,* 19, 4, 413-422.

Kane, R., Oslander, J. & Abrass, I. (1989). *Essentials of Clinical Geriatrics.* (2nd ed.) New York: McGraw-Hill, Information Services Co.

Kaplan, R.M., Sallis, J.F. & Patterson, T. L. (1993). *Health and Human Behavior.* New York: McGraw-Hill, Inc.

King, A.C., Blair, N., Bild, D.E., Dishman, R.K., Dubbert, P.M., Marcus, B.H., Oldridge, N.B., Paffenbarger, R.S.,

Powell, K.E. & Yeager, K.K. (1992). Determinants of physical activity and interventions in adults. *Medicine and Science in Sports and Exercise,* 24, 6, S221-S235.

Kogan, N. (1990). Personality in aging. In J.E. Birren & K.W. Schaie (Eds.) *Handbook of the Psychology of Aging.* (3rd ed). San Diego: Academic Press.

Lesnoff-Caravaglia, G. (Ed.) (1987). *Handbook of Applied Gerontology.* New York, N.Y.: Human Sciences Press, Inc.

Lewis, C.B. & Campanelli, L.C. (1990). *Health Promotion & Exercise for Older Adults: An Instructor's Guide.* Rockville, Md.: Aspen Publishers, Inc.

Marcus, B.H. & Stanton, A.L. (1993). Evaluation of relapse prevention and reinforcement interventions to promote exercise adherence in sedentary females. *Research Quarterly for Exercise and Sport,* 64, 447-452.

Markus, B.H. & Owen, N. (1992). Motivational readiness, self-efficacy and decision-making for exercise. *Journal of Applied Social Psychology,* 22, 3-16.

Markus, B.H., Rakowski, W. & Rossi, J.S. (1992). Assessing motivational readiness and decision-making for exercise. *Health Psychology,* 11, 4, 257-261.

Marlatt, G.A. & Gordon, J.R. (1985). *Relapse Prevention: Maintenance Strategies in Addictive Behavior Change.* New York: Guilford Press.

Marlatt, G.A. & Gordon, J.R. (1980). Determinants of relapse: Implications for the maintenance of behavior change. In P.O. Davidson & S.M. Davidson (Eds.) *Behavioral Medicine: Changing Health Lifestyles* (410-452). Elmsford, N.Y.: Guilford Press.

Myers, G.C. (1990). Demography of aging. In R.H. Binstock & L. K. George (Eds.) *Handbook of Aging and the Social Sciences.* (3rd ed). San Diego, Calif.: Academic Press.

Ostrow, A.C. (1984). *Physical Activity and the Older Adult: Psychological Perspectives.* Princeton, N.J.: Princeton Book Co.

Prochaska, J.O. & DiClemente, C.C. (1983). Stages and processes of self-change of smoking: Toward an integrative model. *Journal of Consulting and Clinical Psychology,* 51, 390-395.

Prochaska, J.O. & DiClemente, C.C. (1982). Transtheoretical therapy: Toward a more integrative model of change. *Psychotherapy: Theory, Research, and Practice,* 20, 161-173.

Salthouse, T. (1990). *Theoretical Perspectives on Cognitive Aging.* Hillsdale, NJ: Lawrence Erlbaum Associates.

Sonstroem, R.J. & Morgan, W.P. (1989). Exercise and self-esteem: Rationale and model. *Medicine and Science in Sports and Exercise,* 21, 329-337.

Spirduso, W. & MacRae, P.G. (1990). Motor performance and aging. In J. Birren, J. Lubbon, J. Cichowlas Rowe & D. Deutchman (Eds.) *Handbook of the Psychology of Aging.* (3rd ed). San Diego, Calif.: Academic Press.

Spotts, H.E., Jr. & Schewe, C.D. (1989). Communicating with the elderly consumer: The growing health care challenge. *Journal of Health Care Marketing,* 9, 3, 36-44.

Stephens, T. & Craig, C. (1990). *The Well-being of Canadians.* Ottawa, Ontario: Canadian Fitness and Lifestyle Research Institute.

Steuart, G.W. (1993). Social and behavioral change strategies. *Health Education Quarterly,* (Supplement 1), 113-135.

U.S. Department of Health and Human Services. (1996). *Physical Activity and Health: A Report of the Surgeon General.* Atlanta, GA: U.S. Department of Health and Human Services, Centers for Disease Control and Prevention, National Center for Chronic Disease Prevention and Health Promotion and The President's Council on Physical Fitness and Sports.

Viney, L.L., Benjamin, I.Y.N. & Preston, C.A. (1988). Promoting independence in the elderly: The role of psychological, social and physical constraints. *Clinical Gerontologist,* 8, 3-17.

Wankel, L.M. (1987). Enhancing motivation for involvement in voluntary exercise programs. In M.L. Maehr (Ed.) *Advances in Motivation and Achievement: Enhancing Motivation* (vol. 5). Greenwich, Conn.: JAI Press.

Ward, P.J. & Preziosi, R.C. (1994). Fostering the effectiveness of groups at work. In J.W. Pfeiffer (Ed.) *The 1994 Annual*

Developing Human Resources San Diego, Calif.: Pfeiffer and Company.

Willis, J.D. & Campbell, L.F. (1992). *Exercise Psychology.* Champaign, Ill.: Human Kinetics.

Wood, J.B. (1989). Communicating with older adults in health care settings: Cultural and ethnic considerations. (Special Issue: Developing leadership in geriatric education.). *Educational Gerontology,* 15, 4, 351-362.

Suggested Readings

On social issues and aging:

Dychtwald, K. (1989). *Age Wave: The Challenges and Opportunities of an Aging America.* Los Angeles: Jeremy Tarcher Inc.

On aging and health:

Ferrini, A.F., & Ferrini, R.L. (1993). *Health in the Later Years* (2nd ed.). Dubuque, Iowa: William C. Brown.

On research, theories and behavior change skills for physical activity for all ages:

Willis, J.D. & Campbell, L.F. (1992). *Exercise Psychology.* Champaign, Ill.: Human Kinetics.

U.S. Department of Health and Human Services. (1996). *Physical Activity and Health: A Report of the Surgeon General.* Atlanta, GA: U.S. Department of Health and Human Services, Centers for Disease Control and Prevention, National Center for Chronic Disease Prevention and Health Promotion and The President's Council on Physical Fitness and Sports.

common health challenges faced

BY OLDER ADULTS

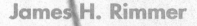

James H. Rimmer

James H. Rimmer, Ph.D., is an associate professor in the Department of Disability and Human Development at the University of Illinois, Chicago. Dr. Rimmer has been directing exercise clinics for older adults since 1981. He is currently the project director of the Center on Health Promotion Research for Persons with Disabilities, which is funded by the Centers for Disease Control and Prevention.

The fastest growing segment of adults older than 65 is comprised of those older than 85 (Rimmer, 1994). This remarkable extension of life brings with it the reality that most older adults will have to live for years, maybe even decades, with one or more chronic conditions. However, though these conditions limit the ability of older adults to exercise, they should not be a deterrent to physical activity. Adults now entering their seventh and eighth decades of life have heard for the last quarter century that exercise is one of the most important aspects of a healthy lifestyle. As a result, many are continuing to participate in physical activity well into their 70s, 80s and even 90s.

Clearly, despite the number of chronic health problems that an elderly person acquires in later life, exercise can and should be an integral part of maintaining and, in some cases, improving their functional mobility. Research demonstrates that persons with chronic conditions such as arthritis or diabetes can improve their physical function by engaging in regular physical activity (Rimmer, Braddock & Pitetti, 1996).

Older adults with heart disease or osteoporosis also can improve their health by choosing to remain physically active (Lewis & Bottomley, 1994), and regular physical activity can positively impact many other chronic conditions (Rimmer, 1994).

Given this demographic shift toward an older, more frail population, fitness professionals must understand the major types of chronic conditions that affect the elderly, and be able to develop safe and effective exercise programs for this clientele. This chapter presents the chronic conditions most commonly experienced by older adults, and discusses guidelines for developing exercise programs that address them.

The Development of Health Problems in the Elderly

Lawrence and Jette (1996) developed a model to describe what they refer to as the disablement process. According to their model, disability and health problems among the elderly occur with several rapid changes in an individual's life.

During the first stage, *pathology*, a disorder such as rheumatoid arthritis or osteoporosis enters the person's life and causes an *impairment*. Impairments can be classified as both anatomical (i.e., bone loss) and structural (i.e., muscle atrophy) in nature, and often lead to a *functional limitation* that causes a restriction in certain physical or mental tasks (i.e., difficulty walking). If the individual does not reverse this process through exercise and rehabilitation, the functional limitation usually worsens, resulting in a *disability*. During this final stage, the individual is unable to perform certain essential movements, such as dressing, walking, getting in and out of a bathtub, climbing steps, etc., and depends more on others for care. The loss of physical mobility often sets off a spiral of depression and failing health.

Your role as a fitness professional is to prevent older adults with chronic health conditions from entering the *impairment* or *functional limitation* stages by incorporating exercise into their lifestyles. Exercise can slow the decline in physical function by preventing further deterioration and, in some instances, by improving the individual's functional mobility.

The goal of an exercise program for older persons with chronic health conditions is not to eliminate the disorder, but to increase the person's fitness level so they are able to maintain as much physical independence as possible. For example, an exercise program for a person with rheumatoid arthritis is not aimed at eliminating the condition, but rather at improving their ability to perform activities of daily living (ADLs), giving them greater control over their environment.

Major Chronic Health Problems Experienced by Older Adults

Several age-related medical conditions affect the elderly that can be divided into six categories: cardiovascular, respiratory, musculoskeletal, metabolic, neurological and sensory (see Table 3.1).

Cardiovascular Disorders

Heart disease is the No. 1 killer of Americans and the most common cause of death among the elderly (Abrams, Beers & Berkow, 1995). While nearly every older adult has an element of heart disease, recent medical advances allow more and more individuals with advanced coronary heart disease to live longer.

Table 3.1

Chronic Conditions Often Experienced by Older Adults

Cardiovascular	Respiratory	Musculoskeletal
Heart disease	Asthma	Osteoarthritis
Hypertension	COPD	Rheumatoid arthritis
		Low-back pain

Metabolic	Neurological	Sensory
Diabetes	Parkinson disease	Visual disorders
Obesity	Alzheimer disease	Auditory disorders

Coronary Artery Disease

Coronary artery disease (CAD) is the primary type of heart disease experienced by older adults. As a person ages, fatty plaque forms inside the arterial walls and causes the arteries to become narrow or blocked. Consequently, blood flow to the myocardium (heart muscle) is reduced. This process is known as **atherosclerosis,** a condition that causes the artery walls to become narrow and brittle. When the arteries become almost completely blocked, the person may experience a heart attack (myocardial infarction), irregular heart rhythm or congestive heart failure.

Other cardiovascular complications include hypertension (high blood pressure), pump failure, valvular problems and peripheral vascular disease (atherosclerosis in the legs). Any of these conditions make the heart less effective in pumping blood to the working muscles, and should be considered when developing exercise programs for older clients.

Symptoms

An early symptom of coronary artery disease is **angina pectoris** (chest pain or discomfort), but it is less common in older adults than in younger persons. More common symptoms of coronary artery disease in older individuals include **dyspnea** (difficulty breathing), diminished exercise tolerance, chronic fatigue and disorders of the heart rhythm, which may cause **syncope** (faintness), **paresthesia** (tingling sensation) and confusion. Electrocardiographic findings are similar to those found in younger persons with CAD (Abrams, Beers & Berkow, 1995).

Developing a Safe Exercise Program

A cardiac rehabilitation program administered under the guidance of a physician, nurse and/or exercise specialist is the safest exercise environment for a person with known coronary artery disease. However, there may come a point when both the client and physician decide that a fitness center is an acceptable place to exercise. If an older adult with coronary artery disease wants to exercise under your guidance, it is imperative to make certain that the exercise regimen is safe for them. Request a specific exercise prescription from the client's physician, and do not alter the program without written approval. Adhere to the following safety concerns when working with clients with coronary artery disease:

Reduce physical exertion. Be aware of the signs of heart distress (chest pain, irregular pulse, difficulty breathing, dizziness), and make sure the client does not exhibit any of these symptoms while exercising. If these symptoms do appear, stop the exercise immediately and notify the client's doctor. Always keep emergency telephone numbers on file in case a client needs immediate medical attention. Clients who are symptomatic during exercise should move into a Phase II or Phase III cardiac-rehabilitation program where they will be monitored closely.

Avoid exposure to extreme heat or cold. As a person ages, their body becomes more sensitive to heat and cold, and it is more difficult to retain or dissipate heat. Maintain a comfortable temperature and humidity level inside the exercise room, and avoid extreme hot or cold temperatures. Frequent water breaks and adequate ventilation are two ways to avoid temperature-induced problems.

Mitigate emotional stress. Emotional stress is a marker for heart problems. If your client exhibits early signs of depression, or you notice a personality change, there may be new sources of stress in their life. This could exacerbate a heart condition or predispose them to new problems. The loss of a spouse or close friend, for example, can be a tremendous hardship. If your client is experiencing more stress than usual, reduce exercise intensity and spend a few extra minutes with them. Weekly three- or four-minute phone calls during these difficult times may enhance your relationship with your client.

Discourage consumption of large meals before exercise. Older adults should never exercise after eating a large meal. Some studies suggest that consumption of a large meal could trigger a heart attack in an older client with advanced coronary artery disease. If combined with exercise, large meal consumption may put clients at an even higher risk. Always check to make sure your older clients do not exercise sooner than one hour (ideally closer to two hours) after a meal.

Exercise Guidelines

1. Because it may be impractical to have every older adult with heart disease perform a stress test before beginning an exercise program, a physician's written consent should be in each older client's file. The consent should indicate that the client's heart condition will not complicate the exercise regimen you develop. Adhere to the exercise prescription and do not alter it in any way unless written approval is given by the physician.

2. Make sure that the client has taken their heart medication before each exercise session and always check their heart rate and blood pressure before beginning activity. If the client's blood pressure is significantly higher than normal (usually more than 20 mmHg for the systolic reading), do not allow them to exercise that day. Take blood pressure readings before, during and after exercise to ensure that there are no major cardiovascular changes occurring during the session.

3. Use the Rating of Perceived Exertion (RPE) scale to gauge exercise intensity in clients who are taking beta blockers, a heart medication that blunts the heart-rate response to exercise. You may have to teach the client how to measure RPE to ensure accuracy.

4. Individualized exercise programs are recommended for persons with cardiovascular disease because group activities usually do not allow the attention that is required to monitor a client's vital signs (i.e., blood pressure, heart rate, respiration, skin color, RPE, general feelings). Though a physician-prescribed program is the safest method, your client may prefer group exercise. Their physician must give written approval for a program that includes group exercise, and may recommend activities that can be performed within a specified intensity level.

Hypertension

Hypertension is a cardiovascular problem for 50 percent of Americans over age 65 (Abrams, Beers & Berkow, 1995). It has been coined the silent killer because half the people who have hypertension are unaware of it. There is a strong relationship between hypertension and coronary artery disease, stroke, congestive heart failure and peripheral vascular disease (Lueckenotte, 1996).

According to the Fifth Report of the Joint National Committee on Detection, Evaluation and Treatment of High Blood Pressure (1993), hypertension is defined as a systolic blood pressure greater than 140 mmHg and a diastolic pressure greater than 90 mmHg. One of the more common hypertension conditions among older persons is isolated systolic hypertension, which is defined as a systolic pressure of greater than 160 mmHg and a diastolic pressure less than 90 mmHg. Several clinical studies have shown that an elevated systolic blood pressure is a better predictor of cardiovascular complications than an elevated diastolic blood pressure. Moreover, people with isolated systolic hypertension are much more likely to die of heart failure or stroke (Abrams, Beers & Berkow, 1995).

Symptoms

Most people with mild to moderate hypertension do not exhibit any symptoms, but those with severe hypertension may experience headaches, fatigue, dizziness and heart palpitations.

Exercise Guidelines

1. The American College of Sports Medicine (1995) recommends a pre-exercise screening and assessment before developing an exercise program for persons with hypertension. Since there are other factors to consider in older clients with hypertension (i.e., age, number of chronic conditions, medication), their physician should provide specific guidelines for exercise intensity, frequency and duration.

2. Persons with a systolic blood pressure greater than 180 mmHg or a diastolic blood pressure greater than 110 mmHg should not begin an exercise program until drug therapy has been initiated (Goldberg & Elliot, 1994). Participation in an exercise program should only begin once the medication has controlled the hypertension and the person does not experience any side effects.

3. Use RPE to monitor exercise intensity in clients taking beta-blocking drugs. Consult with their physicians to determine the RPE value that should be targeted.

4. Always take the client's pre-exercise blood pressure to ensure they have taken their medication (older persons who have forgotten to take their medication will have an elevated blood pressure). To avoid potential problems, clients should not exercise on days when they have not taken their medication.

5. Do not include isometric exercises in programs for clients with hypertension (Moir, 1988). It is a widely held belief that isometric exercise can cause significant increases in blood pressure.

6. Hypertensive individuals should avoid high-intensity exercise (ACSM, 1995). This is especially true for older clients with hypertension since heart disease progresses significantly faster in seniors than in younger individuals.

7. A weight-training program for clients with limited strength should emphasize a high number of repetitions at a low resistance (ACSM, 1995).

8. Along with the exercise program, encourage clients with hypertension to lose weight (if obese); limit alcohol intake to less than 24 ounces of beer, 8 ounces of wine, or 2 ounces of spirits; reduce sodium intake; stop smoking; and reduce dietary saturated fat and cholesterol (ACSM, 1995).

Respiratory Problems

The three most common respiratory problems in older adults are asthma, bronchitis and emphysema. As a group, these conditions are called **chronic obstructive pulmonary disease (COPD)**, a functional diagnosis given to any pathologic process that decreases the ability of the lungs and bronchi to get air into and out of the lungs (Warden-Tamparo & Lewis, 1989). Respiratory disorders are ranked among the top-10 leading causes of death among older persons; within the last decade their incidence has risen more sharply than the other nine causes (Abrams, Beers & Berkow, 1996).

Asthma

Asthma, which comes from the Greek word meaning *to pant*, is defined as a reversible-obstructive-airway disease in which the airways become narrow, resulting in labored breathing. Three pathological changes simultaneously occur during an asthma attack, making it extremely difficult for the person to breathe:

1. The smooth muscles around the bronchioles, which are the small airway tubes in the lungs, go into spasm, contracting and squeezing the bronchial tubes, and making it difficult for air to enter.

2. Thick secretions of mucus accumulate inside the bronchial tubes, further deteriorating the lungs' ability to get oxygen into the blood.

3. The lining of the bronchial tubes thickens and becomes engorged with blood.

Causes of Asthma

The causes of asthma include everything from allergens (an acquired hypersensitivity to a certain substance) to stress. If a person's asthma is related to a specific allergen, it is called **extrinsic asthma;** if it is not related to a specific allergen, it is called **intrinsic asthma** (Pauls & Reed, 1996). Most people with asthma suffer from a combination of the two.

Allergens. Common allergens include pollen; animal dander; certain types of foods, such as strawberries, nuts and chocolates; food additives, such as

monosodium glutamate; feathers; certain medications, such as aspirin; and dusts and molds.

Chemical Irritants. These include dust, paint, deodorants, perfumes and cigarette smoke. For some, the chlorine found in swimming pools also may be a chemical irritant, and new carpeting may precipitate an asthma episode in others. Identify which clients have asthma and alert them to any changes in the exercise facility that may cause an attack.

Temperature. Cold air is a primary trigger of asthma attacks. Many older individuals with asthma may not want to venture out of their homes during the cold winter months to get to a fitness center.

Psychological and Nervous Stimuli. Emotional outbursts of laughter, crying or screaming can stimulate the vagus nerve, which causes the muscles in the bronchial lining of the lungs to tighten and trigger an attack (Plaut, 1984).

Infection. The increased mucus production caused by sinusitis or influenza further narrows the airways and increases the risk of an attack. Pay close attention to a client with asthma who is recovering from a respiratory infection.

Exercise. Researchers speculate that asthma attacks occur during exercise because the temperature in the respiratory passages is lowered and water vapor is removed. This causes a cooling and drying effect in the lungs, which may trigger an asthma attack.

Symptoms of Asthma

Shortness of Breath. The major symptom of asthma is shortness of breath. This uncomfortable feeling has been described as trying to breathe through a pinched straw, and can be an extremely fearful experience for older adults.

Coughing. Persons with asthma may experience a great deal of coughing, particularly during the winter months when cold air exacerbates their condition. The coughing sometimes is associated with an upper-respiratory infection, which also can trigger an asthma attack.

Wheezing. When the coughing sounds as if it originates in the lungs, and audible vibrations can be heard within the chest, the person is wheezing. The wisping noise that is heard when a person is wheezing is related to air being forced through the mucus-filled air passages in the lungs.

Medications Used to Treat Asthma

Familiarize yourself with the drugs most often used to treat asthma and their common side effects. The following medications are listed by their generic name and are sold by various pharmaceutical companies under different trade names.

Theophylline. One of the most commonly prescribed medicines for asthma, theophylline can be taken in pill or liquid form, and should be ingested with a light snack since it can irritate the lining of the stomach. The most common side effects are nervousness, hyperactivity, stomach upset, nausea, vomiting, loss of appetite and headache (Rund, 1990).

Beta-adrenergic Agents. These are sometimes referred to as beta-agonists. Common types include albuterol, isoproterenol, bitolterol, pirbuterol, metaproterenol and terbutaline sulfate. These medications are usually administered with inhalers, and are prescribed to prevent or control exercise-induced asthma.

Cromolyn Sodium. Asthmatics often use cromolyn sodium as a daily medication, or in place of theophylline if it is not well-tolerated. It is usually administered through an inhaler. Cromolyn sodium will prevent an asthma attack from occurring, but will not reverse an attack once symptoms, such as wheezing, have already started. At that point, a beta-agonist must be inhaled to prevent the attack from getting worse.

Corticosteroids. A newer class of drugs used to treat asthma called corticosteroids are used to treat many conditions, but are particularly helpful for controlling severe asthma. Effective in reducing airflow obstruction by stopping the inflammatory reaction, corticosteroids can be administered as tablets or pills, shots in emergency situations, or with an inhaler for everyday management. Popular corticosteroids include beclomethasone diproprionate, flunisolide and triamcinolone acetonide.

Exercise Guidelines

1. Older adults with asthma need to be involved in a safe, structured exercise program. It's important to pay close attention to the client, particularly during the early stages of the program when the risk of an asthma episode is higher.

2. Some older clients with asthma have difficulty exercising for extended periods of time; short, intermittent bouts of exercise may be more effective than one long bout. The exercise program should consist of five or six one- to two-minute exercise routines, with a one-minute rest between each. Once the client becomes conditioned to the program and is able to tolerate longer periods of activity, progressively increase the duration of exercise.

3. Clients with asthma should rest as often as necessary, particularly during group activities. If the client exhibits any shortness of breath, they should stop the activity and rest until they feel comfortable returning to the group. If the client prefers to do something while they are waiting to rejoin the group, have them perform the breathing exercises described in Tables 3.5 and 3.6.

4. Older persons with asthma should always begin exercising at a very low intensity. Watch for shortness of breath during the initial stages of the program. Once the client increases their conditioning level, gradually increase the intensity as long as there are no asthma

symptoms. Some older clients with asthma may not have any trouble exercising at 60 percent to 75 percent of their age-adjusted maximum heart rate, provided they take their medication before the activity. Other clients with a more severe form of asthma will have difficulty exercising at this intensity.

5. The frequency of exercise can range from three to seven days per week, depending on the client's interest and the severity of the asthma.

6. Much of the research on exercise and asthma indicates that swimming is one of the best exercise modalities for this clientele. The temperature and humidity inside a pool allow airways to remain warm and moist, thus preventing an asthma episode. For older persons who do not like to swim, however, short bouts of exercise using a stair stepper, stationary cycle or rowing machine should be relatively safe. Jogging appears to be one of the biggest triggers for exercise-induced asthma and is only recommended for the person who prefers no other modality. Low-impact aerobic dance may be safe if it is not too strenuous.

7. You must make sure that older adults with asthma take their medication before exercising to prevent the onset of an attack. In addition, clients should always carry their inhalers with them. If asthma symptoms arise during the early stages of the program, reduce the activity to a level that will not excessively elevate the client's heart or breathing rates.

8. Warm-ups and cool-downs are especially important for persons with asthma. Research demonstrates that a 15-minute low-intensity warm-up (i.e., brisk walking, riding a stationary bike) can reduce the incidence of asthma episodes during activity in younger athletes. How this translates into an exercise program for older adults is not known at this time, but it does appear

that a sufficient warm-up allows the respiratory system to slowly adapt to the activity and helps prevent an asthma episode.

9. Any person with asthma who enters a fitness center **must** carry a bronchodilator at all times. Always check to make sure your client has their inhaler with them before they begin exercising (i.e., Proventil, Ventolin), as using it is the only way to reverse an attack.

10. A peak flow meter, a small plastic device that measures how quickly a person expires air from their lungs, is a reliable instrument for determining airflow obstruction before an asthma attack occurs. You should have access to a peak flow meter at the exercise site (these cost about $15 to $25). Measuring peak flow rate (see Table 3.2) before a class or exercise session informs you whether the client can safely exercise on that day. A general guideline is that the exercise program should be modified to avoid an asthma episode if peak flow is less than 15 percent of the normal values for the client (which should be established on good days when the client is free of obstruction). It is a good idea also to measure peak flow after exercise, so that both pre-exercise and post-exercise values may be compared.

11. It is crucial to know what to do when an older client has an asthma attack. Refer to Table 3.3 for specific recommendations.

Bronchitis and Emphysema

Two other types of COPD commonly seen in the elderly are chronic bronchitis and emphysema. Chronic bronchitis is an inflammation of the larger airway tubes in the lungs called the bronchi. This condition causes an irritating and productive cough that lasts up to three months and recurs for at least two consecutive years (Pauls & Reed, 1996). It is often linked to heavy cigarette smoking.

Table 3.2

How to Measure Peak Flow Rate

1. Have the client stand, take a deep breath, and place lips around the cardboard mouthpiece that slides into the peak flow meter.

2. The client should blow as fast and as hard as possible into the peak flow meter.

3. Perform peak flow three times and record the highest score in liters.

4. Perform peak flow during the early stages of the program to obtain baseline values on your client.

Emphysema usually occurs in people between the ages of 60 and 70 years, and is characterized by progressive destruction of the alveoli, the sponge-like tissues in the lungs where the exchange of oxygen and carbon dioxide takes place. It also is linked to heavy cigarette smoking.

Symptoms

The symptoms of these two chronic obstructive pulmonary diseases are similar, and include dyspnea (difficulty breathing), coughing, increased mucus production that can be heard in the chest when coughing and wheezing.

Exercise Guidelines

Before developing an exercise program for a client with COPD, classify the client at one of four levels (Rimmer, 1994). Descriptions of these levels are given in Table 3.4. Since it is highly unlikely that a fitness instructor in a community-based setting will work with clients in levels 3 or 4, these guidelines focus on clients in levels 1 and 2.

1. Always consult with the client's physician and/or a respiratory therapist for ideas and tips on preventing dyspnea during exercise. There is a good possibility that the client may already have undergone some kind of a rehabilitation program, and that there are written reports on the client's physical status that may help you develop a safe and effective program.

2. Measure peak expiratory flow rate (refer to Table 3.2) before and after exercise to determine the effects of the activity on breathing capacity. Some activities may produce better airflow readings than others. Those that cause the lowest amount of dyspnea should be used in the program.

3. The American College of Sports Medicine (1995) recommends that a rating of dyspnea be used to gauge the intensity of exercise in persons with COPD. The dyspnea rating scale goes from 0 to 10 (similar to the Borg RPE scale), and a score of three is an indication that the person is exercising at an

Table 3.3

What to Do If a Client Is Having an Asthma Episode

1. Remove the person from the class or room and bring them to a quiet area of the facility.

2. Place the client in a comfortable position (usually sitting down with the arms placed over a table or chair to "open" up the chest).

3. Encourage the person to breathe deeply and slowly (diaphragmatic breathing).

4. If necessary, use a beta-agonist inhaler (this should be left up to the client).

5. A warm drink may help loosen mucus secretions. Do not allow the client to drink cold beverages since this may cause further tightening of the chest.

6. Seek medical attention if symptoms do not improve in a few minutes.

Table 3.4

Functional Classification of Persons with COPD

Level 1 No basic limitations need be observed. The client is in the early stages of the disease.

Level 2 A moderate impairment exists. Duration of exercise may have to be severely restricted.

Level 3 A severe impairment exists. While exercising, the client may need to be carefully monitored by a medical doctor in a controlled setting, such as a laboratory or hospital where oxygen is available as needed.

Level 4 The client may be in chronic respiratory and cardiac failure and may need oxygen from a tank to survive.

intensity of approximately 50 percent of VO_2 peak. The scores for the dyspnea scale are:

    0.5 - very, very slight

    1   - very slight

    2   - slight

    3   - moderate

    4   - somewhat severe

    5   - severe

    7   - very severe

    10 - very, very severe

Record heart rate along with the dyspnea rating to determine the relationship between the two measures.

4. Emphasize interval training techniques for clients exhibiting a high degree of dyspnea during exercise. Providing short periods of rest (one to two minutes) between exercise bouts (one to five minutes in duration) should reduce dyspnea.

5. Exercises that do not produce huge fluctuations in oxygen cost are safer and more effective for this clientele. High-impact exercises or activities that result in dramatic increases in oxygen cost (i.e., running or walking briskly up a flight of stairs) may cause dyspnea.

6. Each exercise session should be preceded by a 10- to 15-minute warm-up that gradually elevates the client's heart rate. Walking outdoors or on a treadmill at a pace that allows the individual to carry on a conversation is a good warm-up activity.

7. End each exercise session with cool-down activities that include flexibility exercises, relaxation techniques and breathing exercises. *Diaphragmatic breathing* and *pursed-lips breathing* are recommended for persons with COPD. These techniques, described in Tables 3.5 and 3.6, have been shown to increase the amount of air taken in through the damaged tissues of the lungs, and reduce the incidence of dyspnea.

8. Some clients with COPD have a tendency to hyperventilate during exercise. This causes further dyspnea since shallow breathing does not allow oxygen to reach the deepest layers of the lungs where gases are exchanged. If a client has a tendency to hyperventilate, teach them how to breathe correctly using diaphragmatic and pursed-lips breathing while walking, riding a stationary cycle or using an upper-arm ergometer.

9. For muscular endurance activities, incorporate high repetitions at a low resistance to avoid dyspnea. Emphasize smooth, coordinated movements that do not require tremendous variations in breathing rate, as would occur while doing push-ups or pull-ups.

10. Exercise prescriptions may need to be adjusted during the winter months. Respiratory infections and cold temperatures often worsen COPD, and many clients will have to severely curtail their activity during illness or when temperatures drop below freezing. Suggest that

Table 3.5

How to Perform Diaphragmatic Breathing

✓ Have the client lie on their back on a mat.

✓ Have the client place one hand on their chest and the other hand on their stomach.

✓ The client should inhale slowly through the nose.

✓ The aim is to inhale so that only the hand on the stomach moves (elevates); the hand on the chest should remain still. This is an indication that the diaphragm is being used to breathe.

✓ Exhale slowly through pursed lips. The stomach muscles should contract.

✓ Rest and repeat several times.

clients who continue coming to the fitness center during the winter months wear a scarf or surgical mask while traveling to the facility. Breathing in cold air before exercise can precipitate dyspnea.

11. Some clients with COPD (or their spouses) continue to smoke, even though they have been diagnosed with a serious disease. Provide as much information as possible about smoking-cessation techniques, and remind these clients that even second-hand smoke can exacerbate their condition.

12. Be familiar with the warning signs for the cardiorespiratory complications that are listed in Table 3.7. If any of these signs appear during exercise, stop the activity and contact the client's physician for further advice.

13. Consider using an oximeter to record oxygen saturation when working with clients with COPD. This device ensures that the exercise program is not causing an oxygen saturation level that is too low, which could lead to respiratory complications. Most respiratory therapists recommend that oxygen saturation remain above 85 percent during exercise (at rest, oxygen saturation is around 97 percent to 98 percent). If oxygen saturation drops below 85 percent, exercise should be stopped and the client should rest and perform diaphragmatic and pursed-lips breathing before resuming the activity.

Musculoskeletal Conditions

It is rare to find an older person in their 70s or 80s who does not experience joint pain. The most common cause is arthritis. Although there are many different types of arthritis (called a *rheumatic disease*) the two most common types affecting approximately 30 to 40 million Americans are osteoarthritis and rheumatoid arthritis.

Table 3.6

How to Perform Pursed-Lips Breathing

✓ Can be done with diaphragmatic breathing or separately.

✓ Inhale slowly through the nose, keeping the mouth closed.

✓ Pucker the lips as if trying to whistle.

✓ Exhale slowly, blowing the air through the pursed lips.

✓ Exhalation should be at least twice as long as inhalation. Begin with a two-second inhalation and a four-second exhalation.

✓ Rest and repeat several times.

Table 3.7

Warning Signs of Cardiorespiratory Complications in Clients Who Have COPD

✓ dyspnea that gradually worsens

✓ swollen ankles

✓ sudden weight gain

✓ high resting heart rate (over 100 bpm)

Osteoarthritis

Osteoarthritis is sometimes referred to as *degenerative joint disease* or *osteoarthrosis*. Osteoarthrosis means an abnormal condition of the joint, which some arthritis experts say is a more accurate term than arthritis, which means an inflammation of the joint. There is usually little joint inflammation with osteoarthritis. Most of the pain is due to the progressive deterioration of *articular cartilage*, which covers the ends of the bones inside diarthrodial joints.

Pathology

Osteoarthritis usually is divided into two types: *primary osteoarthritis* and *secondary osteoarthritis*. Primary osteoarthiritis, which is of unknown origin, is the most common. Secondary osteoarthritis results from an injury or a mechanical derangement of the joint (Mongan, 1990). The joints most often affected by osteoarthritis are the cervical and lumbar spine, hip, knee and distal joints of the hand (the joints closest to the ends of the fingers).

Osteoarthritis is caused by a deterioration in articular cartilage, normally smooth tissue that allows the ends of the bones to glide without friction. The water content of this cartilage increases, indicating that the collagen that provides its structure is breaking up. The cartilage loses its ability to withstand compressive forces, and starts to fray and develop fissures (clefts) that extend into the bone. These bone fragments are called *osteophytes*, or bone spurs. The deteriorating articular cartilage and the accomodating osteophytes create a great deal of pain for millions of older adults.

Rheumatoid Arthritis

Although rheumatoid arthritis can occur at any time during a person's life, it most often occurs between the ages of 25 and 60. In most instances, rheumatoid arthritis is more disabling than osteoarthritis, and causes greater joint deformity, typically in the hands, wrists, and feet. The most common joints affected are the middle joints of the fingers, the knuckles, wrists and feet.

Pathology

Although much has been learned about rheumatoid arthritis, its exact cause is still unknown. It is classified as an autoimmune disease, which means that the person's immune system attacks healthy tissue and damages the joint (Rimmer, 1994).

Rheumatoid arthritis manifests itself in the synovial tissue that lines the outside of the joint, and progresses to an erosion of articular cartilage and bone. In severe cases, the tendons and occasionally the muscles that surround the joint also may become inflamed.

Symptoms

Many of the symptoms and treatment strategies for osteoarthritis and rheumatoid arthritis are similar.

Pain. Many people equate the pain of arthritis to a nagging, dull toothache. Pain caused by rheumatoid arthritis is symmetrical, or bilateral, meaning that both joints are affected. The pain of osteoarthritis is often asymmetrical, meaning that only one joint is affected, although it is not uncommon for both joints to be impacted. Clients who have a high tolerance for pain are able to participate in more activity.

Decreased Range of Motion. Another common symptom of arthritis is decreased range of motion. Sometimes this occurs because of a shortening of muscle fibers associated with inactivity; other times it is due to joint destruction. A client may try to protect the joint by becoming inactive, causing further shortening of the muscle fibers.

Joint Instability. The afflicted joint often becomes unstable as a result of overstretching the supportive ligaments that protect it. This occurs more often with rheumatoid arthritis than osteoarthritis.

Muscle Weakness. Muscle weakness is common in older adults with arthritis because they often think that they protect the joint by not exercising. On the contrary, a lack of physical activity leads to other physical problems and can worsen the symptoms of arthritis.

Diminished Endurance. Just as muscle weakness occurs as a result of inactivity, cardiovascular endurance is lower in sedentary persons with arthritis. Many individuals with arthritis do not understand the value of maintaining good cardiovascular endurance, and think that exercise will do more harm than good.

Classifying People with Arthritis

People with arthritis represent a diverse group. The classification criteria shown in Table 3.8 is a useful guide in determining what type of exercise program best meets the needs of your clients. You will be able to develop a more challenging program for clients in Classes 1 and 2, but may have to work closely with a physical therapist to develop a safe program for clients in Classes 3 and 4.

Exercise Guidelines

Hochberg et al. (1995) note that exercise is a cornerstone of therapy for persons with arthritis. No matter how severe the condition, it is extremely important for older clients with arthritis to participate in physical-activity programs since a deterioration in fitness will clearly worsen their condition. People with arthritis who are deconditioned lose strength, flexibility and endurance, components needed to overcome the pain and physical limitations associated with this disease.

Flexibility

People reluctant to move a painful joint experience extreme tightness in the muscles, ligaments and tendons that surround it. Although protecting the joint from further injury is important, immobilizing the joint may do more harm than good by increasing the tightness/stiffness in and around it. Therefore, flexibility exercises are an essential component of the exercise program for an older-adult client with arthritis.

Follow these general guidelines when developing a flexibility program:

✓ Discontinue flexibility exercises that cause immediate pain, or pain that develops within 24 to 48 hours after exercise.

✓ Teach clients to distinguish between soreness and pain. Soreness occurs when sedentary people begin an exercise program, and is usually located in the muscle. Pain originates in the joint and indicates that the client may have exercised that joint too strenuously. Soreness will ease after the first few weeks of the program, but pain will last longer than a few weeks and may result in further joint damage.

✓ Warming the tissues that surround the affected joint may make the exercise feel more tolerable. Try using hydrocollator pads, which come in different sizes and shapes to fit different joints (i.e., shoulder, knee, ankle), to warm the tissue. Some clients enjoy having the joint warmed before starting the exercise

Table 3.8

Classifying Clients with Arthritis Based on Severity of the Condition

Class 1   Complete ability to carry on all usual duties without a high level of pain or discomfort

Class 2   Adequate ability for normal activities despite the handicap, discomfort or limited motion at one or more joints

Class 3   Ability limited to little or none of the duties of usual occupation or self-care

Class 4   Totally incapacitated, bedridden or confined to a wheelchair, little or no self-care

program, while others do not. Hayes (1996) also notes that some clients may prefer ice to decrease joint pain.

✓ Each of your clients has an individual threshold for holding a static stretch. Some will be able to hold a stretch for six to eight seconds, others longer.

✓ Make sure flexibility exercises are executed correctly, and do not allow the client to bounce during the stretch.

Strength Exercises

It is a misconception that strength exercises will do more harm than good for clients with arthritis. Several studies have documented that strength exercises help people to better cope with their arthritis by improving muscle function and reducing the load on the joint (Feldmann, 1996). Furthermore, arthritic joints that are strength trained improve functional mobility.

Follow these general strength-training guidelines for older adults with arthritis:

✓ Excessive weight training can cause an inflammatory response that results in pain and reduced mobility. Therefore, make sure the client experiences no pain (discomfort or soreness is acceptable, but there should be no pain) during the activity.

✓ If the joints are severely damaged, isometric exercise may be the preferred method of conditioning. Several researchers have noted that isometric activity does not cause inflammation or pain (Basmajian, 1987). Contractions should last approximately six to eight

seconds and be performed two to three times for each muscle group. Isometric exercises can be done with or without weights, depending on the client's initial levels of strength.

Cardiovascular Endurance

Clearly, the best cardiovascular exercise for a client with arthritis is one that does not cause pain. People who have arthritis have successfully used water exercise for years. Some fitness facilities, including the YMCA, even have their own arthritis swim programs. The pool temperature is elevated close to 90 degrees and participants perform different exercises in the water. (Note: The pool also can be used to develop flexibility and strength.)

Cardiovascular equipment that can be used by most arthritic clients without causing high levels of pain includes the arm ergometer (particularly for clients who have knee or hip arthritis), stationary cycle and recumbent stepper. These machines do not excessively overload the joints and can usually be used for several minutes without pain. The Schwinn Air-Dyne ergometer may be a popular choice because clients can use their arms and legs to propel it. This reduces the load on their hip and knee joints.

Follow these general guidelines for improving the cardiovascular endurance of older clients with arthritis:

✓ Use smooth, repetitive motions, such as those used in swimming, cycling and walking.

✓ Jogging or other jarring activities, such as high-impact aerobics, are contraindicated for this clientele.

✓ Use interval training or circuit training routines with clients who are unable to tolerate continuous activity. For example, a client might spend one minute on the bicycle ergometer, followed by a 30-second rest, and then another minute on the ergometer. The client may do this for five or 10 minutes and then move to a new machine that uses different joints, such as the arm ergometer.

✓ Keep the intensity level within the client's comfort zone. The duration and frequency of exercise is more important than the intensity. Encourage 60-minute exercise sessions that allow the client to take periodic breaks. They may be actually exercising for only 30 minutes, but still need a full 60 minutes to incorporate rest periods.

✓ A client with rheumatoid arthritis may occasionally have an acute flareup. This is called an exacerbation, which means that the arthritis has worsened. This has nothing to do with the exercise program, but is part of the disease's progression. The client will probably not be able to exercise during an exacerbation and may have to rest until the symptoms subside.

✓ Clients with arthritis will often fatigue easily. This may be due to a number of problems, including a low fitness level, side effects from certain medications, and not sleeping well at night. Make sure that you do not cause excessive fatigue during the early stages of the program when the client is at high risk for dropping out.

Low-back Pain

Low-back pain is a common complaint among individuals of all ages, but may become a chronic problem for older persons who also have arthritis.

In fact, some low-back pain in older persons may be a direct consequence of osteoarthritis in the spine or another type of rheumatic condition, such as fibromyalgia (Pauls & Reed, 1996). Low-back pain usually is classified as either acute or chronic. Acute back pain is present less than three months and is frequently associated with sciatica or back-related leg pain (Oldridge & Stoll, 1997). Symptoms often clear within three days to six weeks when treated with rest and anti-inflammatory drugs (Plowman, 1992). Chronic back pain lasts longer than three months and treatment includes exercise. However, it is important to consider secondary conditions (i.e., arthritis, fibromyalgia, coronary heart disease) when designing an exercise program.

Exercise Guidelines

Exercises for acute low-back pain should be developed by the client's physician or possibly a physical therapist. However, once the client is cleared to return to full physical activity, you can play an important role in preventing another occurrence of low-back pain.

1. A major goal of an exercise program for persons with chronic low-back pain is to prevent deconditioning. The person may avoid movement for fear of re-injuring the back; in the interim, the muscles weaken and the low back loses some of its extensibility.

2. The exercise program must remain within the client's pain threshold and should not exacerbate any underlying conditions. Sharp pain may be an indication that the exercise is harmful to the condition.

3. Aerobic exercise that puts minimal stress on the back may help to maintain cardiorespiratory endurance. A recumbent bike may be a good modality for mitigating low-back pain in some clients. Check with each client to determine

which type of exercise produces the least amount of pain or discomfort.

4. Strength and flexibility exercises may be helpful for some clients with low-back pain. Their physician or physical therapist may be able to provide you with an established regimen of strength and flexibility exercise for the low back.

Metabolic Disorders

The three most common metabolic conditions seen in elderly adults are diabetes, obesity and osteoporosis. There are more than 50 million Americans who are either overweight or have diabetes, and when you add that number to the millions of older Americans who suffer from osteoporosis, it becomes clear that metabolic disorders are the most prevalent and costly conditions in our society. Obesity and diabetes often are seen in the same individual, since 80 percent of people who have non-insulin-dependent diabetes also are overweight (Franz & Norstrom, 1990).

Diabetes

There are two types of diabetes: Type I, or insulin-dependent diabetes, and Type II, or non-insulin-dependent diabetes. Type I diabetes is the more serious condition and requires daily insulin shots to control blood glucose levels.

Exercise, combined with a proper diet for Type II clients, and insulin and a proper diet for Type I clients, can aid in keeping blood glucose levels under control. However, certain guidelines must be followed to avoid complications.

Exercise Guidelines

1. The intensity, frequency and duration of exercise will depend to a large extent on the severity of the diabetes and the client's initial fitness level. In general, emphasize frequency and duration over intensity.

2. If a client has Type II diabetes and is overweight, follow these guidelines along with the guidelines recommended for Obesity on pages 90-91.

3. A common side effect of Type I diabetes is foot ulcers. Diabetes causes deterioration in the small blood vessels in the feet, diminishing blood flow to these tissues, and resulting in foot ulcers. Foot ulcers can last several months or longer, and are exacerbated by high-impact exercise, such as jogging or aerobics. Discourage clients with foot problems from participating in weight-bearing, jarring exercises such as jogging or racquet sports.

4. Be aware that clients with Type I diabetes must coordinate insulin shots and food intake with their exercise program. Too much exercise, too much insulin or too little food, can cause glucose levels to drop to a dangerously low level. Exercise should not be initiated when glucose levels are under 100 mg/dl.

5. Your major concern when working with older clients with Type I diabetes should be a condition known as hypoglycemia, or what some experts call an insulin reaction. This is defined as a blood glucose level less than 60 mg/dl. An extremely dangerous situation could develop when blood glucose levels drop below this value. Table 3.9 describes the signs and symptoms of an insulin reaction. Exercising under these conditions is a serious hazard and should be avoided until food is consumed and glucose levels rise above 100 mg/dl. Refer to table 3.10 for guidelines on what to do if a client is having an insulin reaction.

6. You should become familiar with a small, pocket-size device called a glucometer that measures blood glucose levels with the prick of a finger and a drop of blood. When a client is having trouble regulating their glucose level, they should bring a glucometer to the exercise session so that blood glucose

Table 3.9

Symptoms of an Insulin Reaction (Hypoglycemia)

✓ Anxiety, uneasiness

✓ Insomnia

✓ Irritability

✓ Nausea

✓ Extreme hunger

✓ Confusion

✓ Double vision

✓ Sweating, palpitations

✓ Headache

✓ Loss of motor coordination

✓ Pale, moist skin

✓ Strong, rapid pulse

levels can be checked before, during and after the activity. In general, blood glucose levels should remain between 100 mg/dl and 250 mg/dl during an exercise session. If blood glucose levels drop below 100 mg/dl, a small snack (i.e., soft drink, orange juice, Gatorade) should be consumed before the exercise session. Have the client wait 10 to 15 minutes and then check their blood glucose level again to make sure that it is in the suggested range. If blood glucose levels rise above 250 mg/dl, discourage the client from exercising, since activity could cause the blood glucose level to go even higher.

7. Clients who have Type I diabetes and are taking beta blockers for a heart condition have a higher risk for developing hypoglycemia because the drugs mask the symptoms of an insulin reaction.

Obesity

Obesity is a common problem among older populations because older adults often think they need not be as concerned with their weight as younger people. People over age 65 rarely follow diet and exercise programs for weight loss. On the contrary, weight should be a greater concern for older populations because of the higher occurrence of secondary conditions (i.e., hypertension, arthritis, heart disease). In addition, as a person grows older and experiences a decline in strength, balance and cardiovascular endurance, any excess weight makes performing activities of daily living (ADLs) more difficult. For these reasons, weight reduction always should be a goal for any older individual who has been classified as overweight or obese.

Exercise Guidelines

1. Exercising three days per week is a good start for obese clients over the age of 65. As the client adjusts to the program, progressively work up to five days per week, varying the program on alternating days to prevent boredom.

2. The higher the level of obesity, the more difficult it will be to exercise. Start with three 10-minute bouts of exercise that consist of 10 minutes of cardiovascular activity (i.e., stationary cycling), 10 minutes of strength training (i.e., biceps curls and triceps extensions using 5-pound dumbbells), and 10 minutes of flexibility exercises. Add minutes to each area of fitness as the client becomes more capable and comfortable with the program. Provide as much rest as is necessary to prevent premature fatigue.

3. Since the major objective of exercise for obese clients is to keep them moving, intensity should not be a focus of the program. Use RPE to gauge exercise intensity if you would like a general index.

4. Utilize structured exercise programs with obese individuals who have never exercised before.

5. Because many obese adults are self-conscious about their weight, it may be beneficial to hold separate classes for males and females.

6. Exercises that compress the chest cavity may impair breathing in the severely obese. Be sure that chest exercises, such as the bench press, do not cause breathing problems.

7. Weight-bearing activities may be difficult for the novice exerciser who also is obese. Try to incorporate non-weight-bearing activities, such as aquatic exercise, and arm and leg cycling.

8. Obese clients will be more susceptible to injury, fatigue and dehydration because of their excess weight. Because these conditions make them more likely

Table 3.10

What to Do If a Client Is Having an Insulin Reaction

1. Stop the activity immediately.

2. Have the client consume a quickly absorbing carbohydrate, such as fruit juice, jelly beans or soda (do not use diet soda).

3. Have the person sit down and check their blood glucose level with a glucometer.

4. Allow the client to rest and return to normal function.

5. When the client feels better, recheck their blood glucose level again.

6. If the blood glucose level is above 100 mg/dl, and the client feels better, resume activity.

to drop out of the program, do not exercise this clientele too strenuously.

9. If the client is interested in an aerobics program, make sure it is low-impact, low-intensity and performed on a floor that will not excessively load the joints.

10. Do not be too concerned about the client's weight during the early stages of the program. The goal is to keep them in the program. Teach the client that even a 10 percent loss in weight will result in tremendous health benefits.

11. Obese people generally have very low self-esteem, so be generous with praise and encouragement, and never place the client in an uncomfortable situation.

12. Develop mini-lectures on dietary guidelines for this clientele. Without a reduction in calories, an exercise program aimed at weight reduction will probably fail.

Osteoporosis

Osteoporosis is a metabolic bone disease that affects five to 10 million older adults (Warden-Tamparo & Lewis, 1989). It is characterized by a gradual reduction in bone mass, which leads to pain, especially in the back and in weight-bearing bones. Like hypertension, osteoporosis has been referred to as a silent killer because there are frequently no clinical symptoms until a fracture occurs.

Fractures associated with osteoporosis are often seen in the thoracic vertebra (dowager's hump or kyphosis), the neck of the femur and the wrist. Fractures can occur through routine bending, lifting and even coughing. Sometimes the affected bones are so thin that lightly tapping a wrist against a hard surface or sitting down too quickly can cause a fracture (Kane, Ouslander & Abrass, 1994).

Exercise Guidelines

1. The key to managing osteoporosis is prevention through smoking-cessation classes, calcium and estrogen replacement and exercise.

2. Weight-bearing activities increase bone mass. Simply standing for several minutes at a time has been shown to slightly increase bone mass in people with severe osteoporosis.

3. Resistance training within the client's tolerance level must be a major cornerstone of the exercise program. Begin with light weights and progressively add more resistance, provided no pain is experienced.

4. Avoid quick, jarring movements that may precipitate a fall or fracture. Twisting movements and increases in intra-abdominal pressure could cause pain.

5. If a dowager's hump is present, avoid excessive overload of the back.

6. Unsupported flexion at the spine could cause excessive loading of the

lower vertebrae. Be careful when performing any back exercises, and if the client complains of pain, stop the activity.

7. No weight-bearing activities should be performed prior to six to eight weeks after a hip fracture.

Neurological Disorders

Dementia or Alzheimer Disease

As you become more accustomed to working with older clients, you will be exposed to a number of older adults who have memory loss and several different types of cognitive impairments. When a person loses memory and other intellectual capacities (i.e., orientation, attention, calculation, language, motor skills), it is called *dementia*. Approximately 60 percent of the dementia in people older than 65 years of age is attributed to Alzheimer disease (Volicer, Fabiszewski, Rheaume & Lasch, 1988).

Exercise Guidelines
Early Stages of Dementia
1. During the early stages of dementia, the client may forget to come to an exercise session or how to do certain exercises. Be patient, understanding and sensitive to the mental anguish that the person is experiencing. Memory loss is one of the most devastating conditions that older adults may experience during their lifetime. Provide moral support and make regular phone calls to remind them of their exercise class.

2. Depression is common in this clientele and may lead to a higher dropout rate. To prevent clients from dropping out of the program, contact them regularly and make sure their caregivers understand the importance of the exercise program.

3. Replace complex exercise routines with simpler activities, such as walking, stationary cycling and basic stretches.

Free weights, treadmills and other pieces of equipment that require steady control of the body could be dangerous to clients with cognitive disorders.

4. Part of the focus of an exercise program for clients with dementia is keeping them interested. Provide lots of verbal praise and positive reinforcement (i.e., birthday card, phone calls, short letters, client-of-the-week award, etc.) to encourage adherence.

5. The intensity of the exercise program is not as important as the frequency and duration. The preferred frequency is five days per week, preferably at the same time each day, so that the client develops a structured exercise routine. Mornings are typically better than afternoons since the client will be rested in the morning and may experience more agitation and fatigue as the day progresses.

Later Stages of Dementia
1. Clients with Alzheimer disease may sometimes exhibit extreme outbursts of anger and physical aggression. Be aware that this behavior has nothing to do with you or the exercise program. These acts of aggression occur randomly and often will last only a few minutes. If the client disrupts a class, remove them from the group until they calm down. Understand that these outbursts are a symptom of the disease and the client often does not understand what they are saying.

2. Memory loss will become more pronounced during the later stages of a progressive cognitive disorder. When this occurs, the client may have to switch from a group exercise class to individual training sessions.

3. The client's caregiver may need to be present during the exercise program. A person with severe dementia often will not want to be left alone with anyone but the caregiver they are most familiar with.

4. It is important to provide a structured exercise routine with little variation for a client in the later stages of a cognitive disorder. An introduction to new activities may confuse them.

5. Never leave a client with Alzheimer disease alone because they will often wander to other parts of the facility.

6. Playing music from the client's generation during the exercise session will occasionally bring back memories and may be a good way to keep them interested in the program.

Parkinson Disease

Although Parkinson disease can occur in younger populations, it is most often seen in individuals older than 50 (Abrams, Beers & Berkow, 1995). Characterized as a chronic, progressive disease that causes movement and postural problems, the condition is caused by a shortage of a chemical produced by the brain called *dopamine*. Dopamine is responsible for transmitting messages across nerve pathways in the brain. When there is not enough dopamine available for the brain to send these messages, voluntary muscle movement and coordination are affected. Tremor (shaking), muscle rigidity and the loss of postural reflexes also characterize the condition. During the early stages of Parkinson disease, shaking is isolated to the hands. Other symptoms include slowness in ambulation and dressing; difficulty getting out of a chair; shuffling gait; stooped over posture; difficulty in starting movements.

Exercise Guidelines

1. Relaxation techniques appear to be very helpful in reducing tremors (Lewis & Bottomley, 1994). Begin a relaxation class in the supine position and gradually progress to sitting and standing.

2. Flexibility exercises also are an important part of the exercise program. Clients with Parkinson disease will exhibit a great deal of muscle tightness and may need some assistance with flexibility routines.

3. Since balance is a major problem for people with Parkinson disease, take every precaution to assure that the exercise environment is safe and that there is a minimal risk of the client falling. A personal trainer should always be in close contact with the client in case they lose their balance. If the client is participating in group exercise classes, recommend that they hold on to a railing or chair, or sit down during the exercise routine.

4. Clients with Parkinson disease usually have a delay when starting a movement, so allow more time to initiate movements.

5. Balance exercises must be an integral part of the exercise program. Both static and dynamic balance exercises should be incorporated into the routine while sitting and standing.

6. Breathing exercises also are important for persons with Parkinson disease. Teach the client to use diaphragmatic and pursed-lips breathing, and have them practice expiring air (e.g., blowing out candles) to strengthen respiratory muscles.

7. Encourage participation in cardiovascular and strength exercises to prevent secondary conditions, such as osteoporosis and muscle atrophy. Be sure that the machines and equipment selected are safe for a clientele with a high risk of falling.

8. Aquatic exercises will be extremely beneficial to this clientele, and will eliminate the risk of a serious fall while performing strength and balance exercises. However, keep in mind that clients with Parkinson disease may have difficulty dressing and undressing, and may not want to go through this burden in order to swim. Be sure the pool temperature is at least 86 degrees.

The instructional strategies listed in Table 3.11 will help you design a program that will lower the frustration level of clients with neurological disorders, as well as your own.

Visual and Auditory Disorders

When working with clients who have visual and auditory problems, remember that the environment must be safe.

Suggestions for Working with Older Adults with Visual Problems

1. Use brightly colored tape (i.e., hot pink or yellow, depending on the background color) to mark objects above and below eye level. Because many older clients will not have a good vertical range of vision, machines that contain parts higher than the client's head or lower than their knees may be bumped into. Objects left in the middle of the floor have the potential to cause a fall.

2. The display panel on some pieces of exercise equipment may be difficult for clients with visual problems to see. Use brightly colored tape to mark the dials, or make arrows that show the client which button to press to increase or decrease time or intensity.

3. Certain types of exercise machines, such as a treadmill, may be hazardous for clients with poor eyesight. To increase safety, use equipment that requires a sitting position, such as a stationary cycle or a recumbent stepper.

4. Because clients with visual impairments may not be able to clearly see your movements, verbal instructions must be precise. Physically guide the client through the correct movement to make the verbal instructions more clear.

5. Clients with visual impairments often use certain pieces of equipment as markers for where they are located in a room. Inform them if any equipment is moved or rearranged.

Suggestions for Working with Older Adults with Auditory Problems

1. Always face the client when you speak. Some older adults may be able to read lips, and when this is combined with the little hearing they have, they will be better able to follow your instructions.

2. Never eat or chew gum while working with the client, as this will make it difficult to understand your speech.

3. Reduce background noise or move to a quiet area while talking to the client.

4. Keep your hands away from your face. If you block your mouth, a client who can read lips will be unable to understand.

5. Do not shout at the client, but speak with a normal, clear tone. Shouting will distort the sound of your voice.

6. Use visual cues as often as possible and combine them with your verbal instructions. Clients with hearing impairments respond well to visual cues (i.e., pictures of the exercises, demonstrations).

Medications and Exercise

Almost every adult older than 65 is taking one or more medications. Despite the benefits that these drugs provide, there are many side effects that could compromise the client's ability to exercise. Although it is beyond the scope of this chapter to review the hundreds of medications that older adults may be taking, it is important that you become familiar with the most common drugs used by this clientele, and that you understand some of the concerns related to exercise and medication.

Table 3.11

Instructional Strategies for Working with Clients Who Have a Neurological Cognitive Disorder

1. *Make the Exercise Simple and Straightforward.* Don't change the exercise routines on a regular basis because it may frustrate a client with memory loss.

2. *Explain Each Movement Clearly and Frequently.* Many clients with neurological impairments will need a frequent explanation of the activity. They will often forget how to perform certain movements and will need to be reminded regularly. Repetition is very important with this group. It may seem boring to you, but will make the client more successful.

3. *Keep the Exercise Routine Structured.* For some clients with dementia, a structured exercise routine (i.e., same room, same equipment, same music, same professional) may need to be established. New activities or surroundings can be frightening for some clients and will agitate others.

4. *Slow Down All Activities.* Everything will have to be slowed down (i.e., speech, tempo, activity) for some clients with dementia. This is especially true for clients with Parkinson disease.

5. *Touching Is a Double-Edged Sword.* Some clients will like to be touched; others will become agitated. You may try to show a client a correct movement and they may become offended by your touch. Keep track of which clients you can and cannot touch. As a client gets to know you, they may become more willing to be touched by you.

6. *Don't Talk Down to the Client.* Many fitness professionals talk to older clients with a neurological disorder as if they are a child, since some of the behaviors are similar to what may be observed in children. This may offend the client or their caregiver. Always treat them like adults no matter how low-functioning they appear to be.

7. *Always Listen and Be Responsive.* Occasionally, clients with dementia will say something that does not make sense. Instead of laughing or becoming agitated, understand that this is part of the disease process and respond to the client in an appropriate manner.

8. *Do Not Allow Verbal or Physical Abuse.* If a client is verbally or physically abusive to you or other members of a class, understand that although this is part of the disorder, it should not be permitted in your class. Remove the client from the group until they calm down.

Beta Blockers

Beta blockers are drugs used to treat cardiovascular disease, including angina pectoris, hypertension and cardiac arrhythmias. They slow down the heart rate and decrease blood pressure by blocking the catecholamine released from the autonomic nervous system. Common brands include Propranolol (Inderal), Nadolol (Corgard), Atenolol (Tenormin) and Metoprolol (Lopressor).

Exercise Concerns

Beta blockers often cause depression, fatigue and dizziness, thus forcing the client to cut down on exercise. Since the function of a beta blocker is to decrease heart rate, heart-rate measures are not a good indicator of exercise intensity. It is recommended that rating of perceived exertion (RPE) be used to monitor the intensity of exercise for clients taking beta blockers.

Diuretics

Diuretics are used to treat hypertension and congestive heart failure. They increase the excretion of sodium and chloride in the urine, producing diuresis. Blood pressure is decreased through the loss of fluid. Common brands include Furosemide (Lasix), Spironolactone (Aldactone) and Hydrochlorothiazide (Esidrix, Hydrodiuril, Oretic, Thiuretic).

Exercise Concerns

Some older adults who are taking diuretics also have a condition known as *postural hypotension*. Postural hypotension causes a drop in systolic and/or diastolic blood pressure, which could lead to dizziness, lightheadedness or a loss of consciousness that could result in a fall. Since clients who are taking diuretics are removing higher levels of fluid from their body, they may need to go to the bathroom more often. This loss of fluid, combined with exercise, could lead to dehydration. Make sure the client is adequately hydrated after the exercise class by having them drink a couple of glasses of water before they leave the fitness center.

Diuretics also can cause weakness and fatigue by depleting the body of its potassium stores. This condition is called *hypokalemia*. If a client complains of weakness or fatigue and is taking a diuretic, ask them to check with their physician to make sure that they do not have this condition.

Hypnotics and Tranquilizers

Hypnotics and tranquilizers are powerful drugs used to calm or quiet an anxious person. The mechanism of action is not completely known. Common brands include Diazepam (Valium), Chlordiazepoxide (Librium), Oxazepam (Serax), Prazepam (Centrax) and Lorazepam (Ativan).

Exercise Concerns

Hypnotics and tranquilizers calm a person, but also increase drowsiness and make it difficult for the client to exercise. It is probably not a good idea for the client to exercise too soon after taking this type of medication. Some hypnotics and tranquilizers also block sweating, thus increasing body core temperature and the risk of hyperthermia (overheating). Make sure that the client has adequate fluid intake before exercise and does not overheat during or after the exercise session. Intensity and duration of exercise may need to be lowered in clients who overheat too quickly.

Antidepressants

Antidepressants are used to treat depression, a condition that afflicts millions of older Americans. The function of an antidepressant is to block the reuptake of neurotransmitters in the brain so that there is an increase in their concentration. Common brands include Imipramine (Tofranil), Amitriptyline (Amitril, Elavil or Endep), Nortriptyline (Pamelor), Desipramine (Norpramin, Pertofrane) and Doxepin (Adapin, Sinequan). A newer class of antidepressants include Fluoxetine (Prozac), Sertraline (Zoloft), Paroxetene (Paxil) and Venlafaxine (Effexor).

Exercise Concerns

Antidepressants can cause dizziness, weakness and lightheadedness. Therefore, pay close attention to the client to avoid a fall. Antidepressants also may cause the client to have a dry mouth, which exercise could exacerbate. It is important to encourage your client to consume small amounts of water before, during and after the exercise session. The newer class of antidepressants (i.e., Prozac, Zoloft) appear to have less side effects than the older medications.

Analgesics

Analgesics are widely used by millions of older adults to relieve some form of joint pain. The function of an analgesic is to block the pain receptors that lead from the brain to the joint.

Many of these drugs are over-the-counter medicines, while others require a prescription. Common analgesics are aspirin, acetaminophen (Tylenol), ibuprofen (Advil, Motrin), naproxen (Naprosyn) and Fenprofen (Feldene). Aside from aspirin and acetaminophen, the other drugs are classified as non-steroidal anti-inflammatory drugs (NSAIDs).

Exercise Concerns

The side effects of NSAIDs in older adults include indigestion, stomach ulcers, kidney problems and, occasionally, gastrointestinal bleeding. Because exercise causes a shifting in blood distribution from the gastrointestinal tract to the working muscles, you must make sure that indigestion or stomach pain is not worsened by exercise. NSAIDS are relatively safe drugs provided they are not taken in high dosages.

The major side effects of taking drugs such as those listed above include drowsiness, ataxia, confusion, lethargy, slurred speech and memory impairment. All of these could adversely effect an exercise session.

Conclusion

Older adults constitute the fastest growing segment of the population. More and more older persons with chronic conditions are electing to remain physically active. Despite their physical limitations, older adults are interested in quality exercise programs delivered by competent fitness professionals. As a result of these demographic shifts, fitness professionals will emerge as major players in health promotion among older adults in the next century.

For more information on fitness programming for older adults with chronic conditions, contact your local heart association, lung association, diabetes association and arthritis association.

References

Abrams, W.B., Beers, M.H. & Berkow, R. (Eds.) (1995). *Merck Manual of Geriatrics*. Whitehouse Station, N.J.: Merck Research Laboratories.

American College of Sports Medicine. (1995). *ACSM's Guidelines for Exercise Testing and Prescription*. Baltimore: Williams & Wilkins.

Basmajian, J.V. (1987). Therapeutic exercise in the management of rheumatic diseases. *Journal of Rheumatology,* 15 (suppl. 15), 22-25.

Feldmann, S. (1996). Exercise for the person with rheumatoid arthritis. In R. W. Chang (Ed.) *Rehabilitation of Persons with Rheumatoid Arthritis* (pp. 91-102). Gaithersburg, Md.: Aspen.

The Fifth Report of the Joint National Committee on Detection, Evaluation, and Treatment of High Blood Pressure. (1993). *Archives of Internal Medicine,* 153(2), 154-183.

Franz, M.J. & Norstrom, J. (1990). *Actively Staying Healthy: Your Game Plan for Diabetes and Exercise*. Wayzata, Minn.: DCI Publishing.

Goldberg, L. & Elliot, D.L. (1994). *Exercise for Prevention and Treatment of Illness*. Philadelphia: F.A. Davis.

Hayes, K.W. (1996). Heat and cold in the management of rheumatoid arthritis. In R.W. Chang (Ed.) *Rehabilitation of Persons with Rheumatoid Arthritis* (pp. 77-89). Gaithersburg, Md.: Aspen.

Hochberg, M.C., Altman, R.D., Brandt, K.D., Clark, B.M., Dieppe, P.A., Griffin, M.R., et al. (1995). Guidelines for the medical management of osteoarthritis. *Arthritis and Rheumatism,* 38, 1541-1546.

Kane, R.L., Ouslander, J.G. & Abrass, I.B. (1994). *Essentials of Clinical Geriatrics*. New York: McGraw-Hill.

Lawrence, R.H. & Jette, A.M. (1996). Disentangling the disablement process. *Journals of Gerontology,* 51B, S173-S182.

Lewis, C.B. & Bottomley, J.M. (1994). *Geriatric Physical Therapy*. Norwalk, Conn.: Appleton & Lange.

Lueckenotte, A.G. (1996). *Gerontologic Nursing*. St. Louis: Mosby.

Moir, T.W. (1988). Nonischemic cardiovascular disease. In B.A. Franklin, S. Gordon & G.C. Timmis (Eds.), *Exercise in Modern Medicine* (pp. 81-106). Baltimore: Williams & Wilkins.

Mongan, E. (1990). Arthritis and osteoporosis. In B. Kemp, K. Brummel-Smith & J.W. Ramsdell (Eds.), *Geriatric Rehabilitation* (pp. 91-105). Boston: Little Brown.

Oldridge, N.B. & Stoll, J.E. (1997). Low back pain syndrome. In J.L. Durstine (Ed.) *ACSM's Exercise Management for Persons with Chronic Diseases and Disabilities* (pp. 155-160). Champaign, Ill.: Human Kinetics.

Pauls, J.A. & Reed, K.L. (1996). *Quick Reference to Physical Therapy*. Gaithersburg: Aspen.

Plaut, T. (1984). *Children with Asthma: A Manual for Parents*. Amherst, Mass: Pedipress.

Plowman, S.A. (1992). Physical activity, physical fitness, and low back pain. In J.O. Holloszy (Ed.), *Exercise and Sport Science Reviews,* vol. 20, (pp. 221-242). Baltimore, Md.: Williams & Wilkins.

Rimmer, J.H. (1994). *Fitness and Rehabilitation Programs for Special Populations*. Dubuque, Iowa: Brown & Benchmark.

Rimmer, J.H., Braddock, D. & Pitetti, K.H. (1996). Research on physical activity and disability: An emerging national priority. *Medicine and Science in Sports and Exercise,* 28, 1366-1372.

Rund, D.A. (1990). Asthma. *The Physician and Sportsmedicine,* 18, 143-146.

Volicer, L., Fabiszewski, K.J., Rheaume, Y.L. & Lasch, K.E. (1988). *Clinical Management of Alzheimer's Disease*. Rockville, Md.: Aspen.

Warden-Tamparo, C. & Lewis, M. A. (1989). *Diseases of the Human Body*. Philadelphia: F.A. Davis.

PRE-EXERCISE
screening and
fitness assessment

Gregory Welch

Gregory Welch, M.S., is an exercise physiologist and president of SpeciFit™, An Agency of Wellness, in Seal Beach, Calif. As a consultant, Welch primarily focuses on special-needs populations. He is on the advisory board of the Lifespan Wellness Center at California State University, Fullerton, and assists in the development and teaching of a certificate course for exercise specialists working with seniors.

More and more, older adults are urged to get some exercise. Virtually all healthcare professionals advocate some form of physical activity for this special population. But what does a recommendation to get some exercise mean? How does an exercise program begin and what determines if it is adequate and appropriate? It all starts with the development of an exercise program, which is the successful integration of exercise science and behavioral techniques that leads to long-term program compliance and attainment of the individual's goals (ACSM 1995). The FITT principle (Frequency, Intensity, Time and Type) is a clever acronym identifying the components of an exercise program. But how are the questions "How often?" (frequency), "How hard?" (intensity), "How long?" (time/duration) and "Which exercise?" (type) answered? Will an exercise program for an 80-year-old cardiac patient be the same as that of a 60-year-old diabetic who has not exercised a day in his life?

The answers to these questions lie in exercise screening and fitness assessment. Though the exercise program is a vital link to improving the quality of older adults' lives, it may not have a chance to succeed without some form of measurement to determine the individual's current fitness and/or functional status. For this reason, a complete assessment of the older adult is essential for developing adequate and appropriate exercise programming. This chapter provides a comprehensive rationale for determining a prudent assessment protocol and details a wide range of measurement and monitoring methods and tools.

The Beginning

The pre-exercise screening and fitness assessment of any individual, regardless of age, involves the gathering of pertinent information. Preventing or reducing the loss of function as a person grows older is dependent, in part, on the detection and treatment of any physical declines that may be precursors to more serious functional losses (Rikli & Jones, 1997). Anthony (1996) states that the screening process allows you to:

1. Identify medical conditions and/or medications that may place the client at risk when participating in certain activities.
2. Discover possible contraindicated activities.
3. Design an appropriate exercise program.
4. Adhere to the legal and ethical requirements of the fitness industry.

Once this information is acquired, the assessment can proceed to the evaluation of the client's functional capabilities. Cotton (1996) suggests using a sound fitness testing battery to evaluate the function of the heart, blood vessels, lungs and muscles according to the physical demands of an individually defined optimal lifestyle. The key to this phrase lies in its latter half. An exercise program should be specific to the physical endeavors of the individual. Similarly, particularly with older adult clients, physical assessments should be specific to each client's needs, abilities and objectives. The benefits of exercise can be measured to the degree that individual limitations are accommodated within exercise training methodology (Williams & Sketch, 1988). This becomes clearer as we attempt to categorize the older adult before beginning the testing process.

Identifying the Older Adult

Chapter 1 of this manual provides excellent information about the physiological effects of aging. Because the aging process is complex, physiology must be the first consideration when working with an older adult client; this consideration is vital in order to proceed with the assessment protocol. Likewise, it is imperative to ascertain both the general characteristics and the specific needs of the elderly (Skinner, 1993).

Chronological Age

No existing single model or paradigm clearly defines the older adult population; rather, a variety of approaches is blended according to individual differences. Because of the relationship between time and the aging process, chronological age is used as an initial identification. The following examples are offered by Spirduso (1995) as simple ways to describe aging: 1) the "young-old" (65-74 years), the "old" (75-84 years), the "old-old" (85-99 years) and the "oldest-old" (>100 years); and 2) sexagenarians (60-69), septuagenarians (70-79), octogenarians (80-89), nonagenarians (90-99) and centenarians (100+). The span of this population is greater than in any other age group, and to label a person as an older adult based solely on age does not give many clues to their fitness level (Evans & Rosenberg, 1991).

Biological Age

Scientists have theorized that biological age is a better tool than chronology when identifying the older adult. Biological aging is the process or group of processes that causes the eventual breakdown of mammalian homeostasis with the passage of time (Spirduso, 1995). It is common to hear someone refer to a person as "young for their age," suggesting that the person apparently has not suffered the decremental effects of biological aging that often accompany chronological age. However, simple observation of a person's appearance provides little more information about a person's functional capacity than chronology.

Because identifying age by outward appearance seems of minimal value, researchers are investigating a biological measurement called a biomarker that is independent of chronological age. This type of measurement has been the focus of gerontologic research for many decades (Mooradian, 1990). Evans and Rosenberg (1991) formulated a list of 10 measurable, modifiable and "vitality-influencing" biomarkers based on a philosophy of maintaining good health for the longest period of time:

1. muscle mass
2. strength
3. basal metabolic rate
4. body-fat percentage
5. aerobic capacity
6. blood-sugar tolerance
7. cholesterol/HDL ratio
8. blood pressure
9. bone density
10. ability to regulate internal body temperature

For assessment purposes, Evans and Rosenberg (1991) suggest that biological age is best calculated on an individual basis. There is, however, a fundamental problem with the biological measurement. Spirduso (1995) states that theories suggesting the existence of a single biological age score assume the existence of a uniform rate of aging across different systems. This criticism is the foundation for the growing interest in biomarkers of aging, including how they are influenced and their potential use for exploring why aging occurs at different rates (Hochschild, 1990). Mooradian (1990) agrees that the rate of aging within a species is quite variable. Furthermore, he states that the availability of biomarkers allows aging rates to be determined on an individual basis, and also allows the impact of various interventions—such as food restriction or exercise—on the aging process to be monitored. By comparing the rates of performance declines in master athletes, Bortz (1996) has suggested that the rate of decline in VO_2max of 0.5 percent per year may be a basic biomarker of the aging process.

The Rate of Aging

The rate of aging is the change in function of organs and systems per unit of time. Under normal circumstances, these changes roughly follow a linear pattern over the life span (Spirduso, 1995). There are, however, a number of factors that confuse what is regarded as normal. Spirduso cites disease, trauma, genetics, nutrition, theories of damage and gradual imbalance, and even gender as factors that affect the rate of deterioration and aging.

There is convincing evidence that physiologic aging advances more rapidly with an accumulation of years of inactivity:

✓ Sedentary individuals have nearly a two-fold faster rate of decline in VO_2max as they age as compared to active individuals (Bruce, 1984).

✓ Muscle mass reduction is primarily responsible for the age-associated loss of strength, which reflects a loss of total muscle protein caused by inactivity, aging or both (Imamura et al., 1983).

✓ The major cause of declining flexibility is a lack of movement in joints not usually used in daily activities (Heath, 1988).

✓ The relative risk of fatal coronary heart disease among the sedentary is about twice that of active individuals (Powell et al., 1987).

✓ Movement times for active people, both young and old, are faster than those in corresponding age groups who are less active (Spirduso, 1975).

✓ Reaction times of older men who have remained active for 20 or more years are equal to or faster than those of inactive men in their 20s (Spirduso, 1975).

✓ Athletes over age 60 have consistently larger-than-expected values for vital capacity, total lung capacity, residual volume, maximum voluntary ventilation and forced expiratory volume based on their body size. The values also are significantly larger than those of sedentary, age-matched, healthy counterparts (Hagberg et al., 1988).

✓ Sedentary living may result in functional capacity losses that are as great as the effects of aging itself (McArdle et al., 1996).

The pre-exercise screening assessment can identify lifestyle behaviors and patterns that are integral to the development of an exercise program.

Activities of Daily Living

Activities of Daily Living (ADL) are the basic tasks of everyday life and independent living, such as eating, bathing and going to the bathroom (Wiener et al., 1990). General measures of health status (i.e., diagnoses or medical conditions) are limited indicators of an individual's independence and functional capabilities (Fillenbaum, 1985). Therefore, researchers have devoted considerable attention to developing health and functional status measures that correspond to practical applications of everyday life as shown in Table 4.1 (Wiener et al., 1990). There are more than 43 different published indexes that assess ADL in both patients and populations (Feinstein et al., 1986).

ADL are classified into three levels of function by the American Geriatrics

Table 4.1

Classification Schema for Elderly Clientele

Level I	Healthy: No major medical problems; in relatively good condition for age; has exercised for the past several years.
Level II	Ambulatory/nonactive: No major medical problems; has never participated in a structured exercise program.
Level III	Ambulatory/disease failure: Diagnosed as having severe coronary artery disease, arthritis, diabetes, or chronic obstructive pulmonary disease.
Level IV	Frail elderly: Relies on partial assistance from professional staff for ADL; can stand or walk short distances (usually less than 100 feet) with an assistive device; spends most of the day sitting.
Level V	Wheelchair-dependent: Relies on total assistance from professional staff for ADL; cannot stand or walk.

Rimmer, J.H. (1994). Fitness and Rehabilitation Programs for Special Populations. *Brown and Benchmark.*

Table 4.2

Hierarchy of Physical Function of the Old (75-85 Years) and Oldest-Old (86-120 Years)

Physically elite

Sports competition
Senior Olympics
High-risk and power
  sports (e.g. hang-
  gliding, weight
  lifting)

Physically fit

Moderate physical
  work
All endurance sports
  and games
Most hobbies

Physically independent

Very light physical
  work
Hobbies (e.g., walk-
  ing, gardening)
Low physical-
  demand activities
  (e.g., golf, social
  dance, handcrafts,
  traveling, automobile
  driving)
Can pass all IADL

Physically frail

Light housekeeping
Food preparation
Grocery shopping
Can pass some IADL,
  all BADL
May be homebound

Physically dependent

Walking
Bathing
Dressing
Eating
Transferring
Needs home or
  institutional care

Disability

Spiduso, W.W. (1995). Physical Dimensions of Aging. *Human Kinetics.*

Society (1989) as basic (BADL), intermediate (IADL) and advanced (AADL)
ADL (see Table 4.2). BADL include the
elemental items of self-care (Katz et al.,
1970). IADL also are referred to as
independent ADL and include tasks
essential to maintaining independence
(Fillenbaum, 1985). AADL are functions well beyond the status necessary
for living alone, and tend to be specific
to each individual. These include recreational, occupational and community-
service functions (American Geriatrics

Society, 1989). ADL measurements are
often used to determine whether an
older adult is capable of living independently. ADL are simple or complex,
depending on the lifestyle history of the
individual. For example, stair climbing
is or is not considered a lifestyle activity,
depending on the person's need to nego-
tiate stairs. Ultimately, as a matter of
lifestyle normalcy, it would be beneficial
to train individuals to climb stairs.
However, in terms of assessment, determining the person's immediate needs

and abilities is the primary objective. Measurement of the activities of daily living is a tremendous tool for answering Spirduso's (1995) question, "What can the older adult actually do?"

The Procedure

The main purposes of exercise testing for the elderly are the same as those for all adults: to define the degree of risk associated with varying work loads, and to establish appropriate intensities for an exercise program (Skinner, 1993). An exercise program should only be developed and used if it is based on sound information obtained from a reliable screening and assessment protocol. Many tests exist to ascertain the information needed to develop an exercise program; you must determine which is most applicable to each client. Skinner (1993) states that not all older people can or should be given exercise tests to determine their fitness level. This is why you must conduct a pre-exercise screening.

Pre-exercise Screening

The pre-exercise screening is the best way to begin gathering information about the older adult's individual needs. A self-reported medical history and an interview enable you to discern the most appropriate exercise-testing protocol.

Medical History and Clearance

Lifestyle behavior, rate of aging and individual differences produce many health issues to consider. Each older adult client should provide a medical history and waiver form prior to beginning any physical assessment procedure. At this time you should completely disclose the risks of an exercise program to your client.

It also is beneficial to acquire a client's physician's consent once an exercise program has been developed. This not only informs the client's physician of the type of exercise the individual will be participating in, but also confirms the validity of the program you have developed and allows the physician to make modifications.

Medication

Be knowledgeable about the various medications that are prescribed for older adults (see Table 4.3). The use and misuse of medication can lead to adverse physical side effects, such as headache, drowsiness, loss of coordination, fatigue, impaired vision and hearing, nausea, irregular heartbeat, orthostatic hypotension, constipation, urinary incontinence, irritability, depression, an inability to concentrate and confusion (Jones 1986). Older adults are more vulnerable to adverse reactions to medication because of the aging process, lifestyle behaviors, acute and chronic diseases, the mixing of drugs, and diet.

Numerous drug regimens are prescribed for a variety of reasons. According to Jones (1986), the most common prescriptive and over-the-counter medications with the greatest risk of adverse effects are:

Prescriptive:

antihypertensive drugs (beta blockers, diuretics)

antiparkinsonism drugs (antidepressants)

psychotropic drugs (sedatives, antianxiety, anticonvulsants, hypnotics, antipsychotics)

Over-the-counter:

aspirin

multivitamins

laxatives

calcium

antacids

antihistamines

Table 4.4

Cardiac Medications: Their Use, Side Effects, and Effects on Exercise Response

Type/Trade Name	Use	Side Effects	Effects on Exercise Response
I. Anti-anginal Agents			
A. Nitroglycerin compounds [*Amyl nitrate; Isordil; Nitrostat*]	Smooth muscle relaxation; decrease cardiac output	Headache, dizziness, hypotension	Hypotension; increase exercise capacity
B. Beta blockers [*Inderal; Propranolol; Lopressor; Corgard; Biocadren*]	Block beta receptors; decrease sympathetic tone; decrease HR, contractility, BP	Bradycardia, heart block, insomnia, nausea, fatigue, weakness, increased cholesterol and blood sugar	Decrease HR; hypotension; decrease cardiac contractility
C. Calcium antagonists [*Verapamil; Nifedipine; Procardia*]	Block influx of calcium; dilate coronary arteries; suppress dysrhythmias	Dizziness, syncope, flushing, hypotension headache, fluid retention	Hypotension
II. Antihypertensive Agents			
A. Diuretics [*Thiazides, Lasix, Aldactone*]	Inhibit NA⁺ and Cl⁻ in kidney; increase excretion of sodium and water and control high BP and fluid retention	Drowsiness, dehydration, electrolyte imbalance; gout, nausea, pain, hearing loss, elevated cholesterol and lipoproteins	Hypotension
B. Vasodilators [*Hydralazine, Captopril, Apresoline, Loniten, Minoxidil*]	Dilate peripheral blood vessels; used in conjunction with diuretics; decrease BP	Increase HR and contractility; headache, drowsiness, nausea, vomiting, diarrhea	
C. Drugs interfering with sympathetic nervous system [*Reserprine, Propranolol, Aldomet, Catapres, Minipress*]	Decrease BP, HR, and cardiac output by dilating blood vessels	Drowsiness, depression, sexual dysfunction, fatigue, dry mouth, stuffy nose, fever, upset stomach, fluid retention, weight gain	Hypotension
III. Digitalis Glycosides, Derivatives [*Digoxin, Lonoxin, Digitoxin*]	Strengthen heart's pumping force and decrease electrical conduction	Arrhythmias, heart block, altered ECG, fatigue, weakness, headache, nausea, vomiting	Increase exercise capacity; increase myocardial contractility
IV. Anticoagulant Agents [*Coumadin, Sodium Heperin, Aspirin, Persantine*]	Prevent blood clot formation	Easy bruising, stomach irritation, joint or abdominal pain, difficulty in swallowing, unexplained swelling, uncontrolled bleeding	
V. Antilipidemic Agents [*Cholestramine, Lopid, Niacin, Atromid-S, Mevacor, Questran Zocor*]	Interfere with lipid metabolism and lower cholesterol and low-density lipoproteins	Nausea, vomiting, diarrhea, constipation, flatulence, abdominal discomfort, glucose intolerance	
VI. Antiarrhythmic Agents [*Cardioquin, Procaine, Quinidine, Lidocaine, Dilantin, Propranolol, Bretylium tosylate, Verapamil*]	Alter conduction patterns throughout the myocardium	Nausea, palpitations, vomiting, rash, insomnia, dizziness, shortness of breath, swollen ankles, coughing up blood, fever, psychosis, impotence	Hypotension; decrease HR; decrease cardiac contractility

McArdle, W.D., Katch, F.I. & Katch, V.L. (1996). Exercise Physiology. (4th ed.) Williams & Wilkins.

Table 4.3

Medications and Substances Affecting Balance

Medications that reduce alertness

- narcotics

- hypnotics

- sedatives

- tranquilizers

- alcohol

Medications that retard central conduction

- narcotics

- hypnotics

- sedatives

- tranquilizers

- analgesics

Medications that impair cerebral perfusion

- vasodilators

- antihypertensives

- some antidepressants

Medications that affect postural control

- diuretics

- digitalis

- some beta blockers

- some antihypertensives

Source: Modified from Professor Bernard Isaacs as cited in appendix A: "A glossary on falls" in Danish Medical Bulletin, Gerontology Special Supplement Series, No. 4: The Prevention of Falls in Later Life: A Report of the Kellogg International Work Group on the Prevention of Falls by the Elderly, 1987.

For additional information about medications for older adults, refer to Chapter 3, the *ACSM Guidelines for Exercise Testing and Prescription* (5th ed.) and the *ACE Personal Trainer Manual.*

The Aging Process and Pharmacokinetics

Pharmacokinetics involve the absorption, distribution, metabolism and excretion of drugs in the human body. Following are five physiological changes that affect the pharmacokinetics of medications in older adults:

Lean body mass decreases as body fat increases. A decrease in lean body tissue and an increase in body fat are due not only to the aging process, but also are partially dependent upon lifestyle behaviors. Body weight rises between the ages of 40 and 60 due to an increase in fat tissue, then declines between the ages of 60 and 80 as lean muscle mass is lost. These changes profoundly affect the distribution and elimination of drugs outside the circulatory system. If a drug must bind to protein tissues, such as acid-organic drugs (diazoxide, digitoxin, penicillin), its distribution is adversely affected by the decrease in muscle mass. When body fat increases, liposoluble drugs, such as barbiturates and psychotropic agents, accumulate in fat tissue and increase the chance of prolonged and toxic effects.

Reduction in total body water. The body consists of about 80 percent water at birth. This figure decreases gradually with age, and it is generally agreed that total body water drops 10 percent to 15 percent between the ages of 30 and 80. Since body water helps dilute water-soluble medications (i.e., diuretics), this decrease in the amount of water in the body lessens the distribution and increases the concentration of these drugs, causing a higher susceptibility to the drugs' toxic effects in older adults.

Decreased efficiency of the gastrointestinal tract. As people age, the efficiency of their gastrointestinal tracts diminishes. Enzyme and glandular secretion, blood flow, gastric motility and sphincter activity decrease, and the effective surface area available for drug absorption is reduced. Thus, the absorption of oral medications in the gastrointestinal tract is slow and less complete. Differences in drug absorption are due to gastrointestinal diseases associated with the aging process, mixing various medications, drug/nutrient interactions and the effects of exercise.

Decreased cardiac output. Reductions in cardiac output decrease blood flow to various body parts. Reduced blood flow to major body organs, such as the liver and kidneys, can result in less efficient drug distribution, metabolism and elimination from the body and, consequently, accumulation and toxicity of drugs taken over an extended period of time.

Decreased efficiency of the liver and kidneys. The liver is the most predominant organ in drug metabolism. As humans age, liver mass diminishes, hepatic blood flow decreases, and fat tends to accumulate in the liver. Combined with other lifestyle abuses, these conditions cause a decline in liver function and a slower, less complete metabolism of drugs. This slower metabolism of drugs—particularly cardiac medications—increases an older adult's vulnerability to adverse effects.

Aging also induces changes in the structure and function of the kidneys. Research has shown that by age 85, kidney mass is about 25 percent less than that of a younger person and renal plasma flow is less than half. These and other changes, such as the build up of fatty tissue, decrease the filtration rate and secretion in the kidneys by about 35 percent over a lifetime and account for a slower removal of drugs.

The Interview

The interview process often is the most comfortable way to begin gathering information and establishing a relationship. A seemingly casual conversation can reveal philosophical and attitudinal biases toward exercise. By having your client describe their past and present experiences with physical activity, whether it be play, sport or occupation, you can gain an overall appreciation of their health status.

Physical Screening

The purpose of a physical evaluation is to identify possible unknown conditions and to establish initial baseline data.

Blood Pressure

The American College of Sports Medicine (1995) considers blood pressure measurement an integral component of the pretest evaluation. Blood pressure is defined as the force of blood distending the arteries and is measured in millimeters of mercury (mmHg). It is determined by cardiac output (CO) and total peripheral resistance (TPR) and, therefore, can be elevated by an increase in either or both (ACSM, 1995).

Blood pressure readings are divided into a top (systolic) and bottom (diastolic) number. The systolic blood pressure represents the maximum pressure created by the heart during ventricular contraction. The diastolic value is the minimum pressure that remains in the arteries during the filling phase of the cardiac cycle, which occurs when the heart relaxes.

A sphygmomanometer and a stethoscope are the tools of blood pressure measurement. The sphygmomanometer consists of a rubber bladder enclosed in a nylon cuff and connected to an inflatable bulb and manometer from which the pressure is read. The stethoscope is used in conjunction with the sphygmomanometer to listen to the sounds made by the vibrations of the vascular walls. These sounds, referred to as Korotkoff sounds, were named after their discoverer in 1905.

Blood pressure assessment can be influenced by client anxiety over unfamiliar surroundings and other stressors, so it may be helpful to let the individual relax quietly for several minutes prior to taking the measurement. With the client seated, place the cuff of the sphygmomanometer around the upper portion of their bare arm, about 1 inch above the crease of the elbow joint. The middle of the bladder should be over the brachial artery on the inner part of the upper arm. Have the client rest their arm comfortably on a table or arm of a chair at heart level. Place the bell of the stethoscope firmly on the brachial artery. You can locate the brachial artery by feeling for a pulse at the inner portion of the elbow joint. Interfering noise, called artifact, can occur if the stethoscope comes in contact with anything during the reading.

While listening to the pulse through the stethoscope, pump the cuff until the pulse disappears. Release the pressure from the cuff at a rate that will cause the pressure to fall about 2 to 3 mmHg per second. If the pressure is released too fast, it will be difficult to obtain an accurate reading. If released too slowly, pressure builds within the arm and causes discomfort and an inaccurate reading. The blood pressure assessment must be performed within 60 seconds to avoid the likelihood of falsely elevated readings. (See Table 4.5 for other potential sources of error in blood pressure assessment.)

As the pressure falls, the Korotkoff sounds can be heard in four or five phases. The first sound represents the systolic blood pressure reading. As the mercury continues to fall, the sound becomes louder and changes to a sharp tapping. This marks the second and third phases, which are not significant. At rest, the fourth and fifth phases usually coincide and involve the disappearance of sound. The point at which the sound disappears is the diastolic reading. During exercise, there may be an audible muffling of the fourth phase; this is the diastolic reading. Because it is not unusual for the vibrations to be heard near zero levels, the fifth phase is not a valid indicator of diastolic pressure (see Table 4.6).

Exercise Response

Systolic blood pressure increases at the onset of exercise due to a rise in cardiac output (Wilmore & Costill, 1994). As exercise intensity increases, the systolic pressure increases linearly (McArdle et al., 1996). Williams (1994) states that a systolic reading above a maximal range of 220 to 240 mmHg is considered a hypertensive response to exercise. A drop in systolic blood pressure (or failure of systolic pressure to increase) that occurs with increased exercise intensity should be viewed as an abnormal test response (ACSM, 1995).

Contrary to the normal rise in systolic blood pressure that occurs during dynamic exercise, diastolic blood pressure should remain constant or decrease by 10 to 20 mmHg as a result of the dilation of the peripheral arterioles of exercising muscle (Williams, 1994). Figure 4.1 illustrates the generalized response for systolic and diastolic blood pressure during continuous, graded treadmill exercise testing.

The ACSM (1995) criteria for contraindicative resting blood pressure for older adults are systolic pressure > 200 mmHg or diastolic pressure > 120 mmHg.

Body Composition

Body composition refers to the overall makeup of the body's total mass. Body composition assessment determines the relative percentages of lean body mass and fat mass.

Sedentary people often boast that their weight is at, or close to, what it was many years before. However, ideal weight, as determined by the bathroom

FIGURE 4.1
Generalized
response for systolic
and diastolic blood
pressure during con-
tinuous, graded
treadmill exercise
testing.

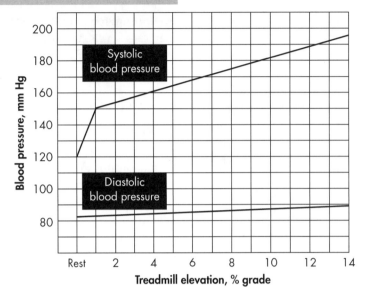

McArdle, Katch & Katch. (1996). Exercise Physiology. Williams & Wilkins.

scale, is a well-rooted misconception that does not consider the relationship between lean body mass and fat mass. In reality, though increases in body weight begin to level off at about age 50 and even begin to decline in the seventh decade, body fat continues to increase (Spirduso, 1995) and lean muscle mass decreases (Stamford, 1988; Muritani, 1981). The loss of lean muscle mass results in an accumulation of body fat (Bemben et al., 1989) and connective tissue (Lexel, 1993). It is clear that a person who maintains their weight without participating in an exercise program to preserve lean muscle tissue is not the picture of health. In fact, excess body fat has been associated with a number of health risks, including heart disease, diabetes, hypertension, arthritis, gall bladder disease, cirrhosis of the liver, hernia, intestinal obstruction and sleep disorders (Cotton, 1996).

There are a variety of methods used to measure body composition. Hydrostatic weighing and skinfold thickness are commonly used with younger populations, but there are notable

Table 4.5

Potential Sources of Error in Blood Pressure Assessment

1. inaccurate sphygmomanometer

2. improper cuff size

3. auditory acuity of technician

4. rate of inflation or deflation of cuff pressure

5. experience of technician

6. reaction time of technician

7. improper stethoscope placement or pressure

8. background noise

9. allowing patient to hold treadmill handrails

10. certain physiological abnormalities, e.g., damaged brachial artery, subclavian steal syndrome, a-v fistula

Table 4.6

Classification of Blood Pressure for Adults Aged 18 Years and Older

Systolic (mmHg)	Diastolic (mmHg)	Category
<130	<85	Normal
130-139	85-89	High Normal
140-159	90-99	Mild (Stage 1) Hypertension
160-179	100-109	Moderate (Stage 2) Hypertension
180-209	110-119	Severe (Stage 3) Hypertension
>210	>120	Very Severe (Stage 4) Hypertension

Fifth Report of the Joint Committee on Detection, Evaluation, and Treatment of High Blood Pressure (JNCV), Archives of Internal Medicine *153: 154-183, 1993*

disadvantages to using these methods with older adults. Hydrostatic weighing (underwater) may make an older individual uneasy as they must be completely submerged in water while the reading is taken. More importantly, while the individual is underwater, they must exhale all the air from their lungs and then wait for a signal before surfacing. This is likely to be *very* uncomfortable for many older adults. In addition, there is a likelihood of gross inaccuracy due to the difficulty of performing the forced expiratory volume (FEV) procedure. It seems safe to say that only a small portion of the older adult population (i.e., the competitive senior) would fare well with this measurement protocol.

The determination of skinfold thickness to measure body composition also is not optimal for older adults. As with hydrostatic weighing, the normative data used to determine the actual percentage of body fat are grouped together in a category listed as 60+ years. This general grouping cannot be considered reliable for a population that is so varied, since, realistically, the senior population potentially spans age 50 and above. Also, the pinching required by this method can create uneasiness and possible pain, and may lead to a negative perception of exercise and program

dropout. The sensitivities and idiosyncracies of the older adult population must always be considered when conducting the physical screening.

You can gain appreciable information about a client's body composition without using such abrasive techniques. Two methods that work well together and are easily performed are body mass index (BMI) and the waist-to-hip ratio.

Body Mass Index (BMI)

The body mass index measures weight in relation to stature, and is calculated by dividing weight (kg) by height (m^2).

Evans and Rosenberg (1991) have listed ideal BMI values for men 60 to 69 years old at 26.6, and 70 to 79 years old at 27. The respective index values for women in the same age categories are 27.3 and 27.8. The researchers also state that figures 20 percent above these ideal values indicate obesity. Spirduso (1995) adds that critical risk factors are associated with extreme BMI values. Very low values indicate a deficiency in muscle mass, whereas very high BMI values suggest excessive fat.

Waist-to-hip Ratio

Waist-to-hip ratio measurements help determine the distribution of fat storage just above and below the waist. The ratio is a simple calculation of the circumference of the waist measured at the level of the navel, divided by the circumference of the hips at the point of greatest protrusion. Men and women have very different ratios that coincide with their gender characteristics. A waist-to-hip ratio below .80 for women and .95 for men is associated with reduced disease risk (Joint Dietary Committee, 1990).

Flexibility

Flexibility is defined as the range of motion around a joint, and is associated with the closeness of the articulating bones and the elasticity of the muscles, ligaments and tendons around the joint (Rimmer, 1994). Normative data for adults over the age of 65 is virtually non-existent and the individual differences are high. Therefore, while standard flexibility exercise assessment protocols are appropriate, measures should only be recorded and periodically checked for progress. Chapter 5 provides a variety of flexibility exercises that you can use in assessing client flexibility.

Tools of the Trade

Baseline data established during the pre-exercise screening and assessment is used to devise the initial exercise program and serves as a standard for the comparison of future results to determine progress. Therefore, continual monitoring of an individual as they exercise is just as important as assessing them at the beginning of the program. This ongoing assessment allows you to: 1) reduce the intensity or curtail the exercise program, 2) maintain the intensity or vary the exercise program or 3) advance the exercise program.

The health history questionnaire, physician's release form and initial interview are important tools to use when beginning the pre-exercise screening portion of the assessment. You should encourage continuous self-reporting to help identify subjective attitudes toward exercise (i.e., enthusiasm, boredom, discomfort and mental and physical fatigue) and to begin to pinpoint possible precursors to injury.

Many of the measuring and monitoring tools and techniques that you use throughout an exercise program can and should be taught to the older adult. Your role as a facilitator of wellness is to educate the individual so they can continue the exercise program autonomously. This is not always as easy as it sounds because the exercise environment is dynamic; by nature, an exercise program is subject to change. An individual must be able to make intelligent decisions based on quality data when dealing with potential changes. Following are the tools and rationale to support the many decisions to be made when assessing and monitoring older adults for an exercise program.

Heart Rate

Heart-rate values are an effective assessment tool. Given their relatively linear relationship to VO_2max, heart-rate measures are a beneficial guide to exercise intensity (ACSM, 1995). A great deal of information can be discerned when heart-rate measures are used in conjunction with the rating of perceived exertion (RPE) scale. Heart rate traditionally has been determined by palpating the pulse for 10 seconds and extrapolating that value over a minute by multiplying by six. Although this method is well accepted, it is highly impractical and, according to Dunbar and Balanos (1996), significantly inaccurate.

For example, heart rates taken during an aerobics class do not represent the work done over the entire class period, regardless of what point they are taken during the class. The pace of an aerobics class can change dramatically or remain constant, depending on the instructor. Although the instructor cannot be expected to control the exertion levels of the entire class, most people believe they do because the instructor chooses the pace of the music and the difficulty of the choreography and provides encouragement throughout the session. And while heart rate indicates whether a participant's pulse is above their training zone, by the time the pulse is found and time is started, 3 to 5 seconds have passed. Add to that the 10 seconds of counting, plus the varying rate of recovery, and you have an imprecise value. If a person does determine that their heart rate is too high, at what point in the workout should they reduce the intensity? This value does not reflect the intensity of the exercise at any previous point during the session.

During a fitness assessment, many cardiovascular testing protocols measure heart rate only at the end of an exercise bout. However, an older adult may take anywhere from 15 to 40 minutes to complete the one-mile walking test, and a great deal of information can be gathered during this time. A heart-rate measurement taken only at the end of the work eliminates a valuable opportunity to collect revealing data. Additionally, because the normative data for evaluating the older adult during this test is unavailable

beyond the seventh decade of life, the information extrapolated from it is of little use. Heart-rate and RPE measurements taken throughout the session could be the only reliable data available. If heart rate is considered an important measurement, then it must be monitored accurately throughout the exercise session with at-a-glance convenience.

Calculating the Training Range

There are two primary methods used to determine heart-rate training range. The first computes the percentage of maximum heart rate (HR max). The second is known as the Karvonen, or heart-rate reserve method. This technique factors in resting heart rate and reflects the percentage of the maximum volume of oxygen (VO_2max). When using the Karvonen method, the percent of heart-rate reserve corresponds to approximately the same percentage of the individual's functional capacity, or VO_2max (ACSM, 1995).

Because true maximum heart-rate values are acquired by using a maximum exercise tolerance test, the constant of 220 minus age will have to suffice when working with older adults. Remember, though, that this common method has a minimum variability of 10 to 12 beats per minute (Durstine & Pate, 1993). The following example illustrates the superiority of the Karvonen method in establishing a training range.

Why not place the power to control workout intensity with the participant? As in any industry, technological advances eventually win out over traditional methods, and it is surprising that wireless telemetry, portable heart monitors have not swept the international fitness community. Use of a portable heart monitor with the RPE scale would give each exercise participant the precise information needed to gauge the intensity of their workout. Furthermore, it would lift the liability burden from the group fitness instructor.

Heart rate example.

Determine the heart rate range from 40 percent to 80 percent for an 75-year-old individual with a resting heart rate of 62 beats per minute.

	220		
–	75		Age
=	145		Maximum Heart Rate
–	62		Resting Heart Rate
=	83		Heart-rate Reserve
X	00.4	X 00.8	Training Heart-rate Reserve
=	33	= 66	
+	62	+ 62	Resting Heart Rate
=	95	= 128	Target Heart-rate Zone

This example clearly illustrates that the training range determined by the heart-rate reserve method is more reliable. The additional data contained in the estimated percent of oxygen consumption is a valuable marker. The ACSM (1995) recommends that the intensity of exercise be 60 percent to 90 percent of HR max, or 50 percent to 85 percent of VO_2max or HR reserve. Many older adults with low initial fitness levels respond to a slow exercise intensity (i.e., 40 percent to 50 percent VO_2max).

Rating of Perceived Exertion (RPE)

In the early 1950s, Gunnar Borg developed the rating of perceived exertion scale to subjectively measure an individual's effort during exercise. The RPE scale has a strong linear relationship to heart rate (Carlton & Rhodes, 1985). Use of this scale can help assess older adult fitness, especially when heart-rate values are not available, such as with cardiac patients taking beta-blockers. Although RPE has been considered an alternative to heart rate, both are uniquely valuable and should be used together when assessing the older adult.

The original scale is a 15-point system that begins at six and ends at 20. A more recent, simplified scale begins at zero and progresses to 10. The terminology used with the revised scale is believed to be better understood by the subject. When using the 15-point scale, values of 12 to 13 (somewhat hard), and 16 (hard) correspond to 50 percent to 74 percent (average of 60 percent), and 85 percent of heart-rate reserve, respectively (ACSM, 1995). The respective values on the Borg 10-point scale are four and six (Skinner, 1993).

Borg (1982) also believed these subjective perceptions carried over to other aspects of measurement. For example, Gordon (1993) has modeled the zero-to-10 scale to reflect the rate of perceived breathlessness (RPB) for patients with breathing disorders. The terminology is similar, but the words "weak" and "strong" on the Borg scale are substituted with "slight" and "severe." In his book on arthritis, Gordon (1993) details a 100-point scale on which individuals rate their perception of pain in each joint.

At SpeciFit, we also use the perceived exertion concept with regard to pain. It may be directly or indirectly related to the physical assessment and can manifest itself in a variety of ways in older adults. Nevertheless, it is important to realize that any physical activity can only continue to the failure of the body's weakest link (Welch, 1996). The solicitation of information about any pain in various parts of the body at discrete points during the session can prevent further injury. For example, a person who is monitored because they are expected to discontinue a walking assessment exercise due to low functional capacity might actually have to quit because of lower leg pain. Conversely, an unmonitored person who experiences discomfort in a quadriceps tendon halfway through the test, but completes the exercise, may begin to establish tendonitis. Even if the pain never becomes significant, it still may induce a negative mindset about exercise and lead to dropout.

The same terminology used in the RPB scale is used to quantify the rate of perceived pain or RPP, also referred to as the weak link index (WLI). The philosophy behind the WLI is the same as that of the RPE, and is pertinent in assessing the older adult.

A zero- to 10-point scale based on the RPE concept to determine the perception of difficulty during a resistance training maneuver may also be used.

This type of measurement is not commonly used because the traditionally accepted method of strength assessment is the repetition-maximum protocol. However, because demanding any form of maximal effort from deconditioned muscle or connective and joint capsular material is unnecessary to establish a fitness program, it is preferable to break from this tradition in the initial assessment and early conditioning of older adults. Jones (1996) developed a one- to five-point scale for similar reasons, stating that controlling the resistance intensity helps to prevent excessive compression and sheer force. An initial test for absolute strength puts the individual at risk of injury and creates a psychological deterrent to exercise. Additionally, the validity of a true test for strength is questionable due to a lack of consideration of the initial stage of neuro-excitation, also known as fiber recruitment.

Therefore, at SpeciFit, we incorporate an additional assessment scale

Table 4.7

Original RPE Scale*		CR10 Scale			Weak Link Index and Rate of Perceived Breathlessness (RPB)		Degree of Difficulty	
6	No exertion at all	0	Nothing at all	"No P"	0	Nothing at all	0	Nothing at all
7	Extremely light	.3			.5	Very, very slight	.5	Very, very easy
8		.5	Extremely weak	Just noticeable	1	Very slight	1	Very easy
9	Very light	1	Very weak		2	Slight	2	Easy
10		1.5			3	Moderate	3	Moderate
11	Light	2	Weak	Light	4	Somewhat severe	4	Somewhat difficult
12		2.5			5	Severe	5	Difficult
13	Somewhat hard	3	Moderate		6		6	
14		4			7	Very severe	7	Very difficult
15	Hard (heavy)	5	Strong	Heavy	8		8	
16		6			9	Very, very severe	9	Very, very difficult
17	Very hard							
18		7	Very strong		10	Maximal	10	Maximal
19	Extremely hard	8						
20	Maximal exertion	9						
		10	**Extremely strong "Max P"**					
		11						
		—						
		•	Absolute maximum Highest possible					

Borg RPE scale © Gunnar Borg, 1970, 1985, 1994, 1998

Borg CR10 scale © Gunnar Borg, 1981, 1982, 1998

* To understand the RPE scale and its administration all users should read: Borg, G. (1998). *Borg's Perceived Exertion and Pain Scales.* Champaign, IL: Human Kinetics.

called the degree of difficulty (DD). When explaining the scale, we ask the individual to set a numeric value on the difficulty of the maneuver. A deconditioned person may have to exert a great deal of effort when lifting the weight of a body part. Monitoring their perception of the difficulty is equally as sensible as monitoring RPE during cardiovascular exercise. After the individual has established a reasonable level of conditioning, a reassessment can include a more aggressive measurement of absolute strength. More detail regarding each of these subjective measurement scales is discussed later in this chapter and in Table 4.7.

The Talk Test

The talk test is another tool used to evaluate an individual during the physical assessment. The ability to engage in conversation during exercise represents work at or near a steady rate (steady state). When the oxygen supply meets demand, a person is able to breathe rhythmically and comfortably. If the work intensity encroaches upon anaerobic metabolism, respirations increase due to an elevation in lactic acid production and the ability to talk diminishes.

Although the talk test is considered somewhat conservative, it is especially useful in assessing the older adult for three reasons:

1. It helps to prevent the individual from working in a potentially at-risk environment.

2. It helps to prevent the psychological deterrent of exhaustion.

3. It helps to ensure the validity of the cardiovascular testing procedure by staving off anaerobic metabolism.

As the client becomes more conditioned, there may be a desire for higher-intensity work, and possibly an interval training protocol (Welch, 1996). However, during the initial stages of

assessment, the talk test maintains a prudent level of work intensity.

Post-exercise Report

To accurately develop an appropriate exercise program and gain an appreciation for the individual's post-assessment perception, there must be follow-up to the initial test phase. The client may be experiencing some level of discomfort or even pain, which can cause them to discontinue an exercise program.

The fact that an individual accomplished a particular amount of work with apparent success does not mean that the level of intensity is appropriate. It is important to discuss the ramifications of the tests with your client one to three days after they have finished the assessment. The information you collect will allow for adjustments if discomfort is experienced due to arthritis, sciatica, lower leg pain, muscle soreness, etc. It is not out of the ordinary for an individual to experience no specific discomfort, but feel completely exhausted. This extended lack of recovery may be due to other lifestyle activities that collectively add to a client's fatigue. It may appear normal, but there is still a potential risk of over-exhaustion.

The post-exercise follow-up also may indicate that the older adult interprets exercise as an interference to their lifestyle. If this occurs, they may be at risk for dropout.

The Art of Assessment

There is an art to the physical assessment of older adults and it lies in an understanding of this unique population. Application of the results of the assessment data yields the most appropriate exercise program and can lead to improved quality of life. It is important to remember that the assessments discussed in this chapter are intended to determine fitness and functional ability levels. There is a vast difference in the overall objective between these field tests and those performed in the clinical environment. Rikli and Jones (1997) state that assessment in the field setting not only needs to be feasible, but socially acceptable as well.

As mentioned at the start of this chapter, for every individual who desires to begin an exercise program, there are a myriad of potential roadblocks that must first be identified. The pre-exercise screening often is taken for granted in younger individuals, but begins the identification process when working with older adults.

Once you have obtained a medical history and physician's waiver and consent, it is time to move on to the next stage, the pre-exercise interview and physical assessment. Because the span of functional ability is so large (from ages 60 to 100+), normative data is yet to be credibly established, and is not used for comparison.

The Pre-exercise Interview

Begin the pre-exercise interview by addressing your client's present level of daily activity. Use questions of frequency, duration and perceived intensity to identify activities of daily living and the extent to which they are carried out. Remember, one person's ceiling is another person's floor; everyone is at some level of activity. You must discover each person's true level before proceeding with further investigation.

Begin with a simple statement that can open a treasure chest of information about the individual's ADL: *Tell me about a typical week in your life.* Ask them to be specific: *Are you still working, or are you retired? If you're working, is any part of your work physical? Can you describe your job? Do you consistently face stairs, ladders, lifting or walking? Do you participate in consistent business activities, such as travel and entertaining, that extend the hours of your work day or week? How do you spend your time away from work? Do you participate in any regular physical activity, recreational travel or physical play? Do you experience any pain during movement?*

If the person is retired, ask what their occupation was. Depending on the answer, the same line of questioning detailed above may be appropriate. Based on how long ago the individual was employed, they may maintain a certain level of fitness due to on-the-job physical training. The contrary also is true regarding a deconditioning level if the individual spent most of their time behind a desk. Ask if they retired by choice or disability. Further questioning after an answer of disability may lead to relevant information specific to the physical assessment: *Have you ever fallen? If so, what were the circumstances? Have there been any other injuries? Did you ever undergo rehabilitation?*

If the individual is not employed, you will need to ask questions about their lifestyle at home. *What does a typical week entail? Who maintains the upkeep of the home, both inside and out? What is the extent of the upkeep?* Try to establish a consistent pattern of physical activity.

Decipher clues about their lifestyle to determine ability and conditioning, whether it is associated with work, or social or recreational activity. For example, if a person reports that the extent of their housecleaning is vacuuming and dusting, this suggests a particular level of ability. If another client reports that their housecleaning involves more ambitious chores, such as mopping floors, cleaning tubs and tile, and washing the windows both inside and out, you can reasonably assume a higher level of ability. A person who can maneuver their body up and down from the floor to mop or clean a tub is likely to have conditioned leg muscles and connective tissue. From a strength standpoint, they also are likely to have a stronger eccentric phase of contraction and are less likely to fall.

Direct questioning about recreational activity can be helpful because it transfers directly to the activities of the physical assessment. Try these questions: *When was the last time you went for a walk? Was it a brisk walk or a stroll? How often do you walk? How far and long do you walk? Do you ever experience pain while walking? If so, where and how long has it been occurring? How long does it take for the pain to subside?* People commonly over-report activity. If this is the case, it will be apparent during the physical assessment.

Physical Assessment

The pre-screening interview is conducted in such detail to determine what physical activity the individual has been engaged in on a regular basis. You must know what they've been doing to determine what they can do. Once this has been established, you can decide the best way to proceed with the physical assessment. A client who has not been consistently climbing stairs, riding a bike or walking the distance you plan to test them at, should not be put through a step test, bike test or distance walking test. Be sensitive to the weak link in the chain (Welch, 1996).

The SpeciFit Walking Test

At SpeciFit, we take the individual for a walk at their desired pace with no pre-established distance. This indirect testing method will yield specific information and is more comfortable for the client. The advantages of eliminating performance anxiety include:

1. Heart rate, RPE, RPB (if applicable) and weak link index (WLI) can be documented throughout the test and used to determine duration.

2. The distance and time initially reported by the individual can be verified.

3. The client's gait pattern and any difficulty negotiating obstacles can be observed.

The parameters of this walking test are common, but the approach appears to be unique. Use the information about walking habits that was gathered in the pre-screening interview as a preliminary guideline and begin the walk. The heart-rate range should be predetermined using the heart-rate reserve method. The individual should wear a portable heart-rate monitor while you hold the display portion. As the walk progresses, engage the client in casual conversation, making inquiries every two to three minutes about their RPE and WLI. Record all information. Remember to let the individual set the pace. RPE and WLI take precedence over heart rate, but all three, plus the comparative time or distance (if applicable), should be continuously evaluated to determine the endpoint of the test. At SpeciFit, RPE is maintained at <6; heart rate at <70 percent HRR; total time does not exceed 10 minutes; and the WLI is maintained at <2 for weight-bearing body parts.

A certain amount of latitude in determining an endpoint is granted if the individual is within their self-reported distance and/or is agreeing to continue. However, a false sense of present conditioning is possible if the client is driven by motivation. This doesn't mean they are unable, just that they are not at a particular level of physical conditioning that will allow them to tolerate an increase without risk of injury. It is more important to assess what the older adult can do successfully than what they can do maximally.

It is necessary to obtain a post-exercise report to complete the walking test.

This simple conversation should take place one to three days after the test to allow the client to report any out-of-the-ordinary pain, discomfort or fatigue. Use the interview to differentiate any problems related to the assessment from any that occur regularly. Do not try to diagnose a particular problem, but identify any concern that could 1) lead to a greater problem should exercise continue; 2) represent the need to reduce the intensity should exercise continue; 3) be necessary cause for referral to an appropriate healthcare professional.

Assessment of Functional Strength and Ability

Although walking is a common lifestyle activity, it is not always indicative of total-body functional ability. Measurement of functional ability determines what exercise is necessary to maintain and improve ADL. Strength is a vital component of the older adult's functional ability, and is traditionally assessed through a one-repetition maximum (1RM) or extrapolated 1RM. Williams (1994) states that the use of 1RM testing is not recommended in persons with no recent exercise history, especially in the elderly. Other test protocols include lighter resistance and maximum repetitions. Although these traditional methods provide information necessary to the eventual establishment of population-specific normative data, the information is not immediately pertinent for functional assessment. Additionally, maximum testing without a preparatory conditioning phase puts the older adult at greater risk.

When testing functional ability it is helpful to first look at functional mobility (Welch, 1995). The SpeciFit Assessment Method of Functional Strength and Ability bases all resistance training for the older adult around the circuit-style method. The individual is first asked to demonstrate the biomechanical patterns common to lifestyle activities, as well as to emulate patterns similar to the movements used in basic resistance-training exercises (i.e., chest press, rowing, shoulder press, leg extension, leg curl, etc.). Body weight is the only resistance used. These are simple voluntary active range-of-motion (VAROM) movements. By observing this movement in the variety of patterns suggested, you can note any difficulties in mobility that might lead to further problems if resistance is added. As part of his post-rehabilitation assessment procedures, Jones (1996) created a scoring system for range of motion (ROM) and strength in all major joints and muscle groups:

3 Full (completes ROM against gravity)

2 Partial (completes $\frac{1}{2}$ of ROM, or better, against gravity)

1 Limited (unable to complete $\frac{1}{2}$ of ROM against gravity)

0 Unable (unable to perform task)

+ No pain, or pain less than 3 on a scale from 1 to 10, add $\frac{1}{2}$ point

- Pain greater than or equal to 4 on a scale from 1 to 10, subtract $\frac{1}{2}$ point

To establish a resistance protocol, make an informed estimate regarding the amount of resistance to use in each separate exercise. Base your decision on three criteria:

1. Data collected during the pre-exercise interview

2. Notable difficulty in the VAROM assessment

3. An understanding of the biomechanical efficiency of the different joint angles

Free weights are preferable to machines when conducting a functional strength assessment. Observe the strength necessary to lift the weight, as well as the stabilization of the joint by the supporting musculature during the action. The range of resistance is 2 pounds to 15 pounds per dumbbell, depending on the individual and the body part being assessed.

Ask the individual to lift the weight in ranges of three to five, five to seven, and seven to 10 repetitions. These ranges promote a philosophy of programming success and allow you to observe the individual's willingness to work. If the person is asked to perform 10 repetitions, but they can only finish eight, they might feel they have failed. To avoid this feeling of defeat, select a range you are confident they will be able to achieve.

At the end of each exercise on the circuit, ask the participant for a degree of difficulty (DD) rating from zero to 10, based solely on how hard it was to lift the weight. The ideal rating is between four and six. Also ask for a WLI value to monitor any pain during or after the lifting procedure. This WLI value is particularly important if the individual has expressed any undue strain with a contorted body or grimacing face. A WLI value greater than two is enough to

Table 4.8

Tinetti Gait Evaluation*

Initiation of gait after told to "go"	Any hesitancy or multiple attempts to start	=0
	No hesitancy	=1
Step length and height	a) Right swing foot	
	Does not pass left stance foot	=0
	Passes left stance foot with step	=1
	Right foot does not clear floor completely with step	=0
	Right foot completely clears floor	=1
	b) Left swing foot	
	Does not pass right stance foot	=0
	Passes right stance foot with step	=1
	Left foot does not clear floor completely with step	=0
	Left foot completely clears floor	=1
Step symmetry	Right and left step length not equal (estimate)	=0
	Right and left step appear equal	=1
Step continuity	Stopping or discontinuity between steps	=0
	Steps appear continuous	=1
*Path***	Marked deviation	=0
	Mild/moderate deviation or uses walking aid	=1
	Straight without walking aid	=2
Trunk	Marked sway or uses walking aid	=0
	No sway but flexion of knees or back or spreads arms while walking	=1
	No sway, no flexion, no use of arms, and no use of walking aid	=2
Walk stance	Heels apart	=0
	Heels almost touching while walking	=1

*Subject stands with examiner; walks down hallway or across room, first at his usual pace, then back at rapid, but safe pace (using usual walking aid such as cane, walker). Maximum Gait Score is 12.
**Estimate path in relation to floor tiles. Observe excursion of one foot over about 10 feet of the course.

Performance-oriented assessment of mobility problems in elderly patients. Journal of the American Geriatric Society, 34, 119-1260.

curtail the assessment of that particular muscle group. Record all values and conduct a post-exercise report in one to three days. Process the information from this report with previous test results to develop the exercise program.

Tests of Function

Many valuable tests look at real-life function in different ways. Balance, coordination, speed and agility all are

important to maintain and improve the physical wellness of the older adult. You are in a position to assist other healthcare professionals in the assessment of these functions.

Tinetti Gait and Balance Evaluation

Tinetti devised a simple, scored screening scale to detect and quantify

Table 4.9
Tinetti Balance Evaluation*

Sitting balance	Leans or slides in chair	=0
	Steady, safe	=1
Arises	Unable without help	=0
	Able but uses arm to help	=1
	Able without use of arms	=2
Attempts to rise	Unable without help	=0
	Able but requires more than one attempt	=1
	Able to arise with one attempt	=2
Immediate standing balance (first 5 sec)	Unsteady (staggers, moves feet, marked trunk sway)	=0
	Steady but uses walker or cane or grabs other objects for support	=1
	Steady without walker or cane or other support	=2
Standing balance	Unsteady (staggers, moves feet, marked trunk sway	=0
	Steady but wide stance (medial heels more than 5 in. apart)	=1
	Narrow stance without support	=2
Nudged (subject with feet close together, examiner pushes lightly on subject's sternum with palm of hand)		
Eyes closed with feet close together	Unsteady	=0
	Steady	=1
Turning 360 degrees	Discontinuous steps	=0
	Continuous steps	=1
	Unsteady (grabs, staggers)	=0
	Steady	=1
Sitting down	Unsafe (misjudges distance, falls into chair)	=0
	Uses arms or not a smooth motion	=1
	Safe, smooth motion	=2

*Subject is seated in hard armless chair. Maximum Balance Score is 16.

Performance-oriented assessment of mobility problems in elderly patients. Journal of the American Geriatric Society, 34, 119-1260.

problems with gait and balance (see Tables 4.8 and 4.9).

For additional testing information, refer to the Williams-Greene Tests of Physical Motor Function, located in the Appendix of *Physical Dimensions of Aging* by Waneen W. Spirduso, Human Kinetics, 1995. Dr. Williams also may be contacted directly by addressing correspondence to: Harriet G. Williams, Ph.D., The Department of Exercise Science, University of South Carolina, Columbia, S.C., 29208.

Special Considerations

By now it should be obvious that the older adult is a complex entity when it comes to health status. Simply by virtue of their age, they hold the potential for a variety of anomalies. It has been noted that four out of 10 older adults (over 65) have a chronic disorder that may result in a functional limitation (Blocker, 1992).You must be able to identify these and other problems through the pre-exercise screening process. Specific consent from the client's physician should be obtained if a client has any of the conditions discussed in Chapter 3, or any other medical condition that would cause exercise or physical assessment to place them at risk.

Conclusion

Appropriate pre-exercise screening and fitness assessment for the older adult is essential. Beginning an exercise program properly can be the catalyst for an individual's continuance into an autonomous lifestyle behavior. The tools necessary to identify the older adult and to determine the initial exercise program for this special population have been provided in this chapter. Accumulating more data in a non-maximal testing environment will ensure a more specific assessment that is safer for the individual. It is important to consider assessment an ongoing process that involves the dynamic nature of exercise as well as the inevitable process of aging.

References and Suggested Readings

American College of Sports Medicine. (1995). *ACSM's Guidelines for Exercise Testing and Prescription* (5th Ed.) Baltimore: Williams and Wilkins.

American Council on Exercise. (1996). R.T. Cotton (Ed.) *ACE Personal Trainer Manual*. San Diego: American Council on Exercise.

American Geriatrics Society. (1989). Assessment in geriatrics: Of caveats and names. *Journal of the American Geriatrics Society*, 37, 6, 570-572.

Anthony, J. (1996). Health screening. In *ACE Personal Trainer Manual*. (2nd ed.) San Diego: American Council on Exercise.

Bemben, M.G., Kuchera, M., and Bemben, D.A. (1989). Physiological changes related to aging: Implications for health and fitness. *Journal of Osteopathic Sports Medicine*, 3, 15-19.

Blocker, W.P. (1992). Maintaining functional independence by mobilizing the aged. *Geriatrics*, 47, 42-56.

Borg, G.B. (1982). Psychological basis of perceived exertion. *Medicine & Science in Sports & Exercise*, 14, 377-381.

Bortz, W.M. (1996). How fast do we age? Exercise performance over time as a biomarker. *Journal of Gerontology: Medical Sciences,* 51A, 5, 223-225.

Bray, G.A. (1979). Obesity in America. *National Institutes of Health,* 79-359, 6.

Bruce, R.A. (1984). Exercise, functional aerobic capacity and aging: Another viewpoint. *Medicine & Science in Sports & Exercise*, 16, 8.

Carlton, R. & Rhodes, E. (1985). A critical review of the literature on the ratings scales of perceived exertion. *Sports Medicine*, 2, 198-222.

Cartee, G.D. (1994). Aging skeletal muscle: Response to exercise. *Exercise Sport Science Review*, 22, 91.

Charette, S.L., et al. (1991). Muscle hypertrophy response to resistance training in older women. *Journal of Applied Physiology*, 70, 1912.

Cotton, R.T. (1996). Testing and evaluation. In *ACE Personal Trainer Manual.*

(2nd ed.) San Diego: American Council on Exercise.

Cumming, G.R. (1993). Children with heart disease. In *Exercise Testing and Exercise Prescription for Special Cases* (2nd ed.) Philadelphia: Lea & Febiger.

Diesel, W., Noakes, T.D., Swanepoel, C. & Lambert, M. (1990). Isokinetic muscle strength predicts maximum exercise tolerance in renal patients on chronic hemodialysis. *American Journal of Kidney Disease*, 16, 109.

Dunbar, C.C. & Balanos, G.M. (1996). Ten-second pulse palpation does not accurately measure heart rate at rest or during exercise. *Medicine & Science in Sports & Exercise*, 28: S-1090, supplement.

Durstine, L. & Pate, R. (1993). Cardiorespiratory responses to acute exercise. In *ACSM Resource Manual for Guidelines for Exercise Testing and Prescription.* (2nd ed.) Philadelphia: Lea & Febiger.

Evans, W. & Rosenberg, I.H. (1991). *Biomarkers*. New York: Simon & Schuster.

Feinstein, A.R., Josephy, B.R. & Wells, C.K. (1986). Scientific and clinical problems in indexes of functional disability. *Annals of Internal Medicine*, 105, 413-420.

Fifth Report of the Joint Committee on Detection, Evaluation, and Treatment of High Blood Pressure. (1993). *Archives of Internal Medicine*, 153, 154-183.

Fillenbaum, G.G. (1985). Screening the elderly: A brief instrumental activities of daily living measure. *Journal of the American Geriatric Society*, 33, 698.

Gilligan, C., Checovich, M.M. & Smith, E.L. (1993). Osteoporosis. In *Exercise Testing and Exercise Prescription for Special Cases.* (2nd ed.) Philadelphia: Lea & Febiger.

Gordon, N.F. (1993). *Arthritis, Your Complete Exercise Guide*. Champaign: Human Kinetics.

Gordon, N.F. (1993). *Breathing Disorders, Your Complete Exercise Guide*. Champaign: Human Kinetics.

Gordon, N.F. (1993). *Stroke: Your Complete Exercise Guide*. Champaign: Human Kinetics.

Hagberg, J.M., et al. (1988). Metabolic responses to exercise in young and older athletes and sedentary men. *Journal of Applied Physiology*, 65, 900.

Haskell, W.L. & Durstine, J. L. (1993). Coronary artery disease. In *Exercise Testing and Exercise Prescription for Special Cases*. (2nd ed.) Philadelphia: Lea & Febiger.

Heath, G.W. (1988). Exercise programming for the older adult. In *ACSM Resource Manual for Guidelines for Exercise Testing and Prescription*, Philadelphia: Lea & Febiger.

Hochschild, R. (1990). Can an index of aging be constructed for evaluating treatments to retard aging rates? A 2,462-person study. *Journal of Gerontology: Biological Sciences*, 45, 6, 187-214.

Imamura, K., et al. (1983). Human major psoas muscle and scarospinalis muscle in relation to age. *Journal of Gerontology*, 33, 678.

Joint Dietary Guidelines Advisory Committee of the United States, Department of Agriculture, Health, and Human Services. (1990). U.S. Dept. of Agriculture.

Jones, J.C. (1986). Interactionary effects of nutrition, medication and exercise. *Southwest Journal on Aging*, 3, 2, 57-74.

Jones, M. (1996). *PERC Post Rehabilitation Protocol Assessment Manual*. San Leandro: American Academy of Fitness Professionals.

Jones, N.L., Berman, L.B., Bartkiewicz, P.D. & Oldridge, N.B. (1993). Chronic obstructive respiratory disorders. In *Exercise Testing and Exercise Prescription for Special Cases*. (2nd ed.) Philadelphia: Lea & Febiger.

Katz, S., Downs, T.D., Cash, H.R. & Grotz, R.C. (1970). Progress in development of the index of ADL. *Gerontologist*, 10, 20.

Leon, A.S. (1993). Diabetes. In *Exercise Testing and Exercise Prescription for Special Cases*. (2nd ed.) Philadelphia: Lea & Febiger.

Lexel, J. (1993). Aging and human skeletal muscle: observations from Sweden.

Canadian Journal of Applied Physiology, 18, 2, 1993.

McArdle, W.D., Katch, F.I. & Katch, V.L. (1996). *Exercise Physiology*. (4th ed.) Baltimore: Williams & Wilkins.

Mooradian, A.D. (1990). Biomarkers of aging: Do we know what to look for? *Journal of Gerontology: Biological Sciences*, 45, 6 183-186.

Muritani, T. (1981). Training adaptations in the muscles of older men. In *Exercise and Aging: The Scientific Basis*. Hillside: Enslow.

Painter, P. (1993). End-stage renal disease. In *Exercise Testing and Exercise Prescription for Special Cases*. (2nd ed.) Philadelphia: Lea & Febiger.

Painter, P. (1986). Exercise during hemodialysis: Participation rates. *Dialysis Transplant*, 17, 21-26.

Powell, K.E., et al. (1987). Physical activity and the incidence of coronary heart disease. *Annual Review of Public Health*, 8, 253.

Rikli, R.E. & Jones, J.C. (1997). Assessing physical performance in "independent" older adults: Issues and guidelines. *Journal of Aging and Physical Activity*, 5, 244-261.

Rimmer, J.H. (1994). *Fitness and Rehabilitation Programs for Special Populations*. Madison: Brown & Benchmark.

Sannerstedt, R. (1993). Hypertension. In *Exercise Testing and Exercise Prescription for Special Cases*. (2nd ed.) Philadelphia: Lea & Febiger.

Skinner, J.S. (1993). *Exercise Testing and Exercise Prescription for Special Cases*. (2nd ed.) Philadelphia: Lea & Febiger.

Spirduso, W.W. (1995). *Physical Dimensions of Aging*. Champaign: Human Kinetics.

Spirduso, W.W. (1975). Reaction and movement time as a function of age and physical activity level. *Journal of Gerontology*, 30, 435.

Spirduso, W.W. & Clifford, P. (1978). Replication of age and physical activity effects on reaction and movement time. *Journal of Gerontology*, 33, 26.

Stamford, B.A. (1988). Exercise in the elderly. In *Exercise and Sports Sciences Reviews*. New York: Macmillan.

Tinetti, M.E. (1986). Performance-oriented assessment of mobility problems in elderly patients. *Journal of the American Geriatric Society*, 34, 119-226.

Trueblood, P.R. & Rubenstein L.Z. (1991). Assessment of instability and gait in elderly persons. *Comprehensive Therapy*, 17, 8, 20-29.

Welch, G.L. (1996). Interval training for the competitive senior. *The Senior Fitness Bulletin*, 3, 2, 15-23.

Welch, G.L. (1996). Strengthening the weak links. *IDEA Personal Trainer*, 7, 9, 13-16.

Welch, G.L. (1995). Training goals for the older adult. *IDEA Personal Trainer*, 6, 1, 31-34.

Welch, G.L. (1995). Stabilization: An integral part of real life function. *The Senior Fitness Bulletin*, 2, 2, 8-9.

Wiener J.M., Hanley, R.J., Clark, R. & Van Nostrand, J.F. (1990). Measuring the activities of daily living: Comparisons across national surveys. *Journal of Gerontology: Social Sciences*, 45, 6, 229-237.

Williams, M.A. (1994). *Exercise Testing and Training in the Elderly Cardiac Patient.* Champaign: Human Kinetics.

Williams, M.A. & Sketch, M.H. (1988). Guidelines for exercise training of elderly patients following myocardial infarction and coronary bypass graft surgery. *Geriatric Cardiovascular Medicine*, 1, 107-110.

Wilmore, J.H. & Costill, D.L. (1994). *Physiology of Sport and Exercise.* Champaign: Human Kinetics.

OLDER ADULT
exercise techniques

Janie Clark

Janie Clark holds a master's degree in exercise physiology and wellness management. She is the author of Full Life Fitness: A Complete Exercise Program for Mature Adults *and* Seniorcise: A Simple Guide to Fitness for the Elderly and Disabled *and the editor of* Exercise Programming for Older Adults *(Haworth Press, 1996) and the*

quarterly magazine Senior Fitness Bulletin. *Clark also serves on the Coalition to Recommend National Curriculum Standards for Preparing Senior Fitness Instructors and is president of the American Senior Fitness Association (SFA), the international organization for fitness professionals who serve older adults.*

In its most basic context, the term *aging* simply refers to the passage of time. On another level, aging involves complicated processes that contribute to an ultimate decline in function. Complex relationships develop between the aging process itself and individual variables such as history of physical injuries or long-term behaviors involving diet, physical activity, smoking, alcohol consumption and drug use. For these reasons, assumptions regarding "normal," "typical" or "average" individual performance abilities become less viable with increasing age. In fact, the older-adult age group is characterized by dramatic individual differences in functional capacity. For example, whereas one 75-year-old person may be unable to lift a 10-pound bag of groceries or walk around the block without assistance, another may compete successfully in marathons (Gersten, 1991; Spirduso, 1995). Clearly, a "one size fits all" exercise programming approach is inappropriate for this population.

Fortunately, a variety of training options is available to older-adult fitness participants. These include group or solitary walking programs, aerobic exercise classes, chair-seated exercise, personal training, balance training, aquatics, relaxation classes, active pastimes such as gardening or square dancing, or simply integrating more physical activity into one's daily routine.

Choosing Among Forms of Training

There are a number of personal variables to take into account when recommending exercise modes for your older-adult clients, including:

✓ Fitness level

✓ Health status

✓ Level of mobility/physical limitations

✓ Source and degree of motivation

✓ Self-efficacy

✓ Time commitment

✓ Needs/goals

✓ Interests

A careful analysis of these variables will help guide your clients toward forms of exercise that will produce beneficial training effects while, at the same time, providing a satisfying physical activity experience that encourages prolonged compliance and adherence.

How should you determine whether to steer a new older-adult exercise client toward a low-impact aerobics class, a personal-training program, chair-seated activity or some other form of training? Although health status and performance assessment results provide critical direction, the decision also should be based on the client's personal preference. This can be identified during an initial interview process, in which the client's goals and interests are explored. Examples of some potential findings and their indicated actions are discussed below.

✓ Does the client have a strong interest in social opportunities for camaraderie and interaction among others in their age group? Does movement to music appeal to the client's tastes? Does the client indicate confidence in their ability to perform and enjoy group exercise? Based on the client's health history, performance assessments and your personal observations during the interview process, is the client physically capable of successfully participating in an aerobics class? Does the class schedule fit into the client's day-to-day routine? Does the class match the client's training goals? If so, a low-impact aerobics class appears to be a good choice for this client.

✓ Is the client motivated by specific health concerns or performance goals that are best met by individualized attention? Does the client's functional capacity significantly exceed or fall below the performance level achieved in group classes? Is a personal-training regimen consistent with the individual's likes and dislikes? Does the client think that they would enjoy working with exercise machines? When the answer to any of these questions is yes, a personal-training program may be a good choice.

✓ Does the client use a wheelchair, or are they otherwise physically restricted with regard to standing, walking or getting up and down? Has the client expressed any misgivings in connection with the ability to successfully participate in fitness training? For example, is the client concerned about the possibility of falling or not being able to get up from the floor after mat exercises? Is the client obviously frail, obese or disabled? If so, then low-impact aerobics may not initially be a viable option for the individual. Although personal training appears to be an appropriate choice, further questions need to be answered before the client is placed in such a program. For example, does the client prefer a group environment? Will a movement-to-music format prove enjoyable and motivational for this client? If so, a chair-seated exercise class may be the best method of reintroducing the individual to a more active lifestyle.

✓ Does the client have a firm idea of what type of activity they want to try? For example, clients that have had positive experiences in swimming pool classes may want to re-enter a water program. Others may prefer a walking program because they view it as a

non-intimidating form of exercise since it does not require learning new skills. Some may be more inclined to take a relaxation or yoga class. In every case, try to accommodate the wishes of the client, augmenting the desired form of exercise, if necessary, with additional activities to achieve a fully balanced program.

Often, a combination of modes is ideal. For example, aerobics class participants may also benefit by performing strength exercises on selected machines. Group classes might include a combination of standing aerobic work and seated muscle work. Alternatively,

---

Table 5.1

General Older Adult Exercise Safety Guidelines

The following precautions apply to all forms of exercise discussed in this chapter:

✓ Obtain medical clearance to exercise.

✓ Never hold the breath. During strengthening exercises, exhale upon exertion and inhale during the release phase.

✓ Do not strain.

✓ Do not hyperflex (over-bend) or hyperextend (over-stretch) the joints. For example, avoid hyperflexion of the neck during curl-ups, and avoid hyperextension of the elbows during arm exercises.

✓ Do not over-grip hand weights, equipment handles or other exercise accessories.

✓ Discourage a competitive atmosphere in group settings.

✓ Limit overhead arm work.

✓ Teach a neutral spine position.

✓ Avoid excessive vertical loading of the spine (by controlling resistance level and other training variables during strength exercise).

✓ Always provide optimal manual support for the back when bending the upper body in any direction and from any position.

✓ Separately perform moves that involve turning or bending the back, rather than combining the two activities.

✓ Use caution with regard to neck exercise. Do not move the neck quickly; avoid hyperflexion due to excessively low nodding, and hyperextension due to backward tilting of the head.

✓ Modify methods that are not well tolerated. If an exercise causes pain, modify or replace it as necessary. Reduce intensity, duration or frequency levels that are too great.

✓ Implement slow, gradual progression.

✓ Avoid known high-risk activities and techniques (for example, straight-legged sit-ups, the hurdler's stretch, the plow, the full cobra, and any other moves identified as potentially dangerous when evaluated according to the criteria provided in Table 5.2).

✓ Remember to err on the side of safety.

chair aerobics classes might include standing muscle work using the back of the chair for balance support. Accomplished group instructors can supervise chair-seated and standing (or mat-exercising) participants in the same class by teaching chair-seated alternative exercises as needed. Relaxation exercises can be incorporated into the cooldown segments of other types of classes and programs. Balance training can play a part in functional-fitness programming, and elements of both can be utilized in either personal training or group settings.

Practically speaking, older-adult programming formats may incorporate elements from a number of reliable training methods, depending upon the needs and preferences of the individual involved. Examples include:

✓ Cross training (combining or periodically changing exercise modes)

✓ Interval training (alternating periods of relatively high-intensity work with periods of low-intensity work)

✓ Circuit training (interspersing aerobic exercise between strengthening activities)

Such changes in exercise mode may be made for the sake of progression. For example, although some participants must remain in chair classes because of physical limitations, others may eventually graduate to more active classes. Persons who have made muscle-conditioning progress in a class may

---

Table 5.2

Exercise Selection: Evaluating the Advisability of Specific Exercises

Below are pertinent questions to answer when considering whether to conduct a specific exercise activity:

✓ What is the purpose of the exercise? (For example, is the goal to warm up, cool down or accomplish aerobic conditioning, flexibility improvement or muscle strengthening? Is the exercise supposed to engage a particular muscle or muscle group?)

✓ Does the exercise effectively fulfill that purpose? (For example, does the exercise actually work the intended muscle group?)

✓ Is the exercise safe for average asymptomatic participants? (For example, does it produce excessive impact or otherwise place unnecessary stress on any joint? Does it place undue pressure on any body part, or immoderate demands on any body system?)

✓ If not, can the exercise practically be modified to an appropriate form? (For example, straight-legged sit-ups can be altered to achieve an acceptable activity by bending the knees and simply curling the trunk forward; deep squats can be replaced by shallower squats.)

✓ If an unacceptable exercise cannot be modified, with what acceptable activity can it be replaced? (For example, the plow can be replaced by leg hugs to stretch the back, gluteals and hamstrings without distressing the neck.)

✓ Is the exercise safe for the specific individual expected to perform it? (For example, does the participant have any special condition that would preclude performing activities that are deemed safe for others in their age group?)

✓ If not, can the exercise be modified to safely accommodate the participant? (For example, should the range of motion be reduced?)

✓ If an unacceptable exercise cannot be modified to safely meet the needs of an individual with a special condition, with what acceptable activity can it be replaced? (For example, if performing floor push-ups strains a participant's wrists, then a wall push-up might be implemented; if that, too, strains the wrists, then the involved upper body muscles can be conditioned with exercises using dumbbells or strength machines.)

Note: When in doubt regarding the implementation of a specific exercise activity or technique, consult your participant's personal physician.

need to increase their intensity level by moving on to a strength-machine workout. Conversely, persons with weak lower-body musculature may need to start with strength-machine workouts to condition the body before attempting a dance-exercise class.

Variations in mode, which are virtually limitless, also may be made for variety's sake. The goal is to conduct effective programming that promotes the development of a lifelong exercise habit.

For a more in-depth discussion of principles related to matching physical needs and ability levels to appropriate training options, please refer to Chapter 6.

Training Guidelines

Following the principles of mode, frequency, duration, intensity and progression helps safely produce and maintain desired training effects. The following guidelines for aerobic, strength and flexibility training—elements essential to a balanced program—should be applied when conducting the various forms of activity addressed in this chapter. In addition, observe general safety precautions, and analyze the safety and effectiveness of specific exercises or techniques (see Tables 5.1 and 5.2).

Complete programs also address balance/coordination (discussed later in this chapter).

Aerobic Exercise

Cardiovascular exercise is any mode of continuous activity utilizing large muscle groups that is rhythmic and aerobic in nature (ACSM, 1990). For safety reasons, low-impact rather than high-impact modes of aerobic exercise are recommended for older-adult participants (Pollock et al., 1991).

The aerobic exercise training guidelines published by the American College of Sports Medicine (ACSM, 1990), the

---

Table 5.3

Basic Guidelines for Aerobic Exercise Training (General Population)

American College of Sports Medicine

✓ Frequency: 3 to 5 days per week

✓ Intensity: 40 percent to 85 percent VO_2max

✓ Duration: 15 to 60 minutes, continuous

✓ Mode: Aerobic activities

American Heart Association

✓ Frequency: 3 days per week, minimum

✓ Intensity: 50 percent to 60 percent VO_2max

✓ Duration: 30 minutes, minimum

✓ Mode: Aerobic activities/health-promotion activities*

American College of Sports Medicine/Centers for Disease Control and Prevention/Report of the Surgeon General on Physical Activity and Health

✓ Frequency: Daily

✓ Intensity: Moderate

✓ Duration: Accumulate 30 minutes per day

✓ Mode: Health-promotion activities*

* Health-promotion activities may include active tasks, such as raking leaves, or taking part in active leisure pastimes.

American Heart Association (Fletcher et al., 1995), and the Centers for Disease Control and Prevention in conjunction with the ACSM (Pate et al., 1995) are, for the most part, consistent (see Table 5.3). In addition to improving fitness level, increased physical activity is recommended for enhancing quality of life and for reducing general health risks. The recent *Surgeon General's Report on Physical Activity and Health* (U.S. Department of Health and Human Services, 1996) encourages a regular, preferably daily, regimen including 30 to 45 minutes of moderate activity—brisk walking, bicycling or even simply working around the house or yard—to lower the risks of developing coronary heart disease, hypertension, colon cancer and diabetes.

To establish and maintain a training intensity that is both safe and sufficient to produce beneficial physiological effects, the intensity level of aerobic exercise should be regularly monitored by rating of perceived exertion (RPE) and/or by heart-rate count (Borg, 1982; Swart, Pollock & Brechue, 1996). The Karvonen formula can be used to determine working heart-rate goals. The formula calculates training heart-rate range based on heart-rate reserve (HRR), the difference between maximal and resting heart rates. Percentage value using the HRR method is approximately equal to percentage VO_2max (i.e., a 50 percent intensity prescription determined by the HRR method equals about 50 percent VO_2max) (Pollock & Wilmore, 1990). (see Tables 5.4 and 5.5)

For older participants, apply aerobic training principles in a manner that discourages potential orthopedic problems and cardiovascular complications. An intensity level of 30 percent to 75 percent VO_2max (with an RPE of 12 to 14 on the Borg 6-to-20 perceived exertion scale) sustained for 30 to 60 minutes is recommended for older adults (ACSM, 1990; Pollock, Graves, Swart & Lowenthal, 1994; Swart, Pollock & Brechue, 1996). Total quantity of work depends upon duration and intensity, which are inversely related. When energy costs are similar, lower-intensity, longer-duration

---

Table 5.4

Karvonen Formula: Estimating Target Heart-rate Zone According to Beats Per Minute

Formulas should not be used to estimate target heart-rate zones for persons using medications that alter heart rate. (In that case, obtain training intensity parameters from your subject's physician.)

In the following example, target heart-rate zone is calculated for a 65-year-old individual with a resting heart rate of 70 beats per minute. The exerciser will work at a moderate intensity level from 50 percent to 75 percent of maximum heart rate (an appropriate range for the typical asymptomatic older adult).

	220			
–	65			Age
=	155			Maximum Heart Rate
–	70			Resting Heart Rate
=	85			Heart-rate Reserve
X	00.5	X	00.75	Training Heart-rate Range
=	43	=	64	
+	70	+	70	Resting Heart Rate
=	113	=	134	Target Heart-rate Zone

Note: Conducting periodic 10-second pulse counts is a convenient method of monitoring heart rate during aerobic exercise. To determine the desirable 10-second count range, divide the target rate values by 6. In this example, the minimum 10-second count is 19 (113 divided by 6) and the maximum is 22 (134 divided by 6).

Table 5.5

Rating of Perceived Exertion (RPE): A Subjective Method of Monitoring Intensity Level

The Borg 6 to 20 scale*:		A simpler scale preferred by many professionals and participants (4 to 7 represents desirable intensity range):	
6	No exertion at all		
7	Extremely light	1	Very, very light
8		2	Very light
9	Very light	3	Fairly light
10		4	Light
11	Light	5	Somewhat hard
12		6	Moderately hard
13	Somewhat hard	7	Hard
14		8	Very hard
15	Hard (heavy)	9	Very, very hard
16		10	Extremely hard
17	Very hard		
18			
19	Extremely hard		
20	Maximal exertion		

Borg RPE scale © Gunnar Borg, 1970, 1985, 1994, 1998

*To understand the RPE scale and its administration all users should read: Borg, G. (1998). *Borg's Perceived Exertion and Pain Scales.* Champaign, IL: Human Kinetics.

aerobic exercise produces benefits comparable to those achieved through higher-intensity, shorter-duration exercise (Swart, Pollock & Brechue, 1996). For previously sedentary older adults, low- to moderate-intensity exercise of longer duration is generally preferable. Initially, the exerciser's tolerance may limit duration. If so, rest periods between exercise bouts allow the exerciser to achieve the recommended duration. Accumulating the recommended exercise duration through short periods of activity, either within a single workout session or during several sessions throughout the course of a day (Pate et al., 1995), provides significant health benefits (DeBusk, Stenestrand, Sheehan & Haskell, 1990; Paffenbarger, Hyde, Wing & Hsieh, 1986).

A frequency of three to five days per week (spaced throughout the course of the week) is generally recommended (ACSM, 1990). Since low-fit older exercisers may be able to tolerate only very-low-intensity, short-duration (five- to

10-minute) exercise sessions, a slight increase in frequency (four to five days per week) will help meet desirable total energy expenditure levels (approximately 1,000 kcal per week). Research suggests that the health benefits associated with physical activity are related primarily to total quantity of activity, regardless of exercise mode, duration or intensity (ACSM, 1990; Pollock, Graves, Swart & Lowenthal, 1994). In addition to intensity and duration, mode may have a practical impact upon frequency. For example, short- to moderate-duration, low-intensity walking can usually be safely performed seven days per week.

Progression should be implemented slowly. A two- to six-week, low-intensity starting phase permits adaptation with minimal risk for injury. The next phase (lasting approximately six months to a year for middle-aged and elderly participants, respectively) involves gradual progression by conservatively increasing both duration and intensity. Generally, duration can safely be increased by five-minute increments every two weeks for middle-aged participants and every three to four weeks for elderly participants. Intensity can then be adjusted as appropriate. The final phase involves maintaining the desired health/ fitness level. During this stage, current or equivalent training activities are continued with an emphasis on long-term adherence (Pollock, Graves, Swart & Lowenthal, 1994; Swart, Pollock & Brechue, 1996).

Strength Training

A number of influential research projects (Frontera et al., 1988; Fiatarone et al., 1990; Charette et al., 1991; Fiatarone et al., 1994; Westcott, 1995) have been instrumental in formulating current thought on the following optimal strength-training methods.

✓ Intensity: 70 percent to 80 percent of 1 RM (repetition maximum: the maximum amount of resistance a subject can control during one repetition of a given exercise); alternatively, an RPE of 12 to 14

✓ Repetitions: eight to 15

✓ Progression: maintenance of 70 percent to 80 percent 1 RM, reassessed every two to four weeks

✓ Sets: one to three

✓ Speed of movement: six to nine seconds per repetition

✓ Rest: one to three seconds between repetitions; 90 to 120 seconds between sets

✓ Frequency: two to three times per week (with at least 48 hours of rest between sessions)

✓ Range of motion: complete, according to individual tolerance

Keep in mind that 1 RM may be quite low in many older adults. As a result, 70 percent to 80 percent of 1 RM will not necessarily represent what is typically considered heavy resistance. Initially performing three to five repetitions at 60 percent to 80 percent 1 RM may be sufficient for the frail to activate dormant muscle fibers and enhance muscle strength and functional movement (Hyatt, 1996). Learning and mastering new exercise movements without the use of any resistance other than gravity and body weight may initiate progression for low-fit exercisers. In time, low-fit exercisers may graduate to the use of resistive exercise bands, dumbbells and strength machines (Hyatt, 1996).

Flexibility Training

Basic recommended programming parameters (ACSM, 1995; Ettinger, Mitchell & Blair, 1996; Gladwin, 1996) are outlined below:

✓ Mode: static (held) stretching, rather than ballistic (bounced) stretching

✓ Frequency: two to seven days per week

✓ Duration: position held for five to 40 seconds per stretch (depending upon the muscle or muscles being stretched)

✓ Repetitions: one to five per stretch

✓ Intensity: range gently increased in each position until mild muscular tension, but not pain, is experienced

✓ Progression: develop fuller ranges naturally with time and practice

Depending upon time constraints, individualized program goals and the specific stretches undertaken, participants may gradually progress from the lower to the higher ranges of frequency, duration and repetitions provided by the parameters listed above. The lower ranges (for example, two to three days per week frequency) may be employed for maintenance programs, whereas progression to the higher ranges (for example, five to seven days per week frequency) should be gradual to achieve significant increases in range.

Techniques

Only the boundaries of one's creativity limit older-adult fitness programming possibilities. In this regard, there are no effectual substitutes for practice and experience. Because no single publication includes every beneficial exercise, enjoyable dance step or successful combination, fitness professionals must develop and rely upon their own personal skills, talents and resourcefulness. Those faculties can, in turn, be recruited to implement and build upon the specific techniques and model routines provided below.

Warm-up and Cool-down Techniques

Adequate warm-up and cool-down periods are especially important to older adults since, with age, sudden vigorous work or abrupt cessation of strenuous exercise can strain the heart. Warm-up periods of approximately 10 to 15 minutes and post-aerobic cool-down/ stretch periods of approximately 15 minutes are recommended for healthy participants. Beginners and persons with special conditions such as arthritis or cardiovascular problems generally need longer warm-up and cool-down sessions.

In addition to gradually increasing circulation and heart rate, the warm-up should prepare the body for movements that will be required during the workout. All of the major joints and muscles should be gently engaged. The back should be warmed up in a vertical position before lateral spinal movements are performed. As a general rule, resistive devices should not be used during the warm-up. Although mild stretches of the calves, hamstrings, back and other body parts may be performed toward the end of the warm-up, the warm-up should primarily be devoted to continuous rhythmic movements, and intensive stretching should be saved for the cooldown. A thorough warm-up should be completed whether the training to follow is to be aerobic, resistive, stretching, some combination or a total-body workout. These principles apply whether the warm-up is undertaken in a chairseated or standing position, or in a gym or swimming pool. Most standing landbased warm-ups can be adapted to the chair or pool. Treadmill and stationary cycle warm-ups can be augmented by a few minutes of rhythmic movements targeting the upper body. See Table 5.6.

The cool-down period following aerobic exercise should feature sloweddown movements that allow the heart rate to gradually decrease. For this purpose, the warm-up techniques described in Table 5.6 also can be used during the cool-down phase. This type of activity should be continued until pre-aerobic respiration and heart-rate states are

---

Table 5.6

Practical Warm-up Techniques

Provide balance support, such as the wall or the back of a sturdy chair, as necessary.

✓ Perform easy-paced walking and/or marching (on a treadmill, in place, or moving about).

✓ Perform slow, non-strenuous pedaling on a stationary cycle.

✓ Perform relaxed dancing at a conservative tempo (for example, the Charleston, small kicks and toe touches to the front, back or sides).

✓ Perform rhythmic, limbering exercises (for example, heel raises, knee lifts, arm reaches and shoulder lifts and circles) working through a full, pain-free range of motion.

re-established (general rule: until the heart rate descends to fewer than 100 beats per minute). If heart rate remains high despite a lengthy cool-down period, even milder movements should be undertaken until heart rate declines, and the participant should consult his or her physician. Also, in that case, the preceding aerobic work may have been too demanding; extra attention should be paid to monitoring the body's response during future aerobic activity, which should be moderated, if necessary, to help guard against over-exertion. If strength-training exercises have not already been performed during the workout, they can be introduced after the active post-aerobic cool-down: Briefly stretch, then complete the strengthening routine, followed by a few minutes of gently active cool-down activity and sustained stretches involving all of the body's major joints and muscles. If strength-training work was completed prior to the aerobics segment, then the post-aerobic cool-down should proceed to the complete stretch routine. The final cool-down/stretch period is a good time to include balance work and relaxation activities.

As with aerobic exercise, the cool-down period following intensive strength work should include a few minutes of gently active cool-down activity (i.e., walking or slow cycling) prior to sustained stretching activity. This is because the cardiovascular system needs a transition period after any type of strenuous activity (W.L. Westcott, personal communication, January 24, 1997).

Various workout formats require slightly different warm-up and cool-down applications (see Table 5.7).

Chair-seated Exercise Techniques

Along with low-impact aerobics, aquatics and even fitness walking programs, chair-seated exercise classes are particularly conducive to movement-to-music techniques (see Table 5.8).

In muscle-conditioning programs that involve only light (or no) extrinsic resistance, it is not necessary to work the muscle groups in a particular order. For example, the chair-seated, low-impact aerobics and aquatic routines provided later in this chapter generally follow top-to-bottom sequences. Engaging opposing muscles in succession is recommended. As resistance increases, it becomes more important to work larger muscle groups earlier (when participants are less fatigued).

Regarding chair-seated exercise, avoid training people in chairs without some good reason. Weight-bearing activities and movements in active functional positions are generally more effective than chair-seated work. However, as discussed above, there are a number of reasons for having participants exercise in chairs, including issues related to endurance, mobility and self-efficacy. When serving the frailest older-adult populations, seated exercise may be the only practicable method and, in fact, chair exercises may need to be adapted to bed exercise programming for some individuals.

Most chair-exercise instructors prefer to work with chairs that do not have arms. This increases the potential range of movement and makes a broader variety of exercises possible. However, some facilities are already equipped with armchairs when a fitness program begins and the instructor must work with what is available. Likewise, many chair-seated exercisers use wheelchairs. Therefore, it is important to develop the ability to work effectively using arm chairs. During chair exercise, it is critical that support be provided for the participant's back, perhaps by utilizing a pillow, pad or rolled towel if necessary. It is equally important that the participant's feet contact the floor fully, which can be accomplished by using a book, stool or some other type of platform if needed.

Table 5.7

Incorporating Warm-up and Cool-down Phases into Various Workout Formats

Aerobics-only Workout

✓ Warm-up: at least 10 to 15 minutes

✓ Aerobic work: approximately 30 minutes or longer

✓ Active post-aerobic cool-down: at least five to 10 minutes (or longer if needed for heart-rate recovery)

✓ Stretching/relaxation: at least five to 10 minutes, longer if time permits

Muscle Strengthening-only Workout

✓ Warm-up: at least 10 to 15 minutes

✓ Strength training: approximately 30 to 40 minutes*

✓ Stretching/relaxation: at least five to 10 minutes, longer if time permits

Stretch-only Workout

✓ Warm-up: at least 10 to 15 minutes

✓ Stretching/relaxation: approximately 30 to 40 minutes, longer if desired

Total-body Workout with Strength Work Preceding Aerobic Work

✓ Warm-up: at least 10 to 15 minutes

✓ Strength training: approximately 15 minutes*

✓ Brief stretching: approximately two to five minutes

✓ Repeat active rhythmic warm-up activities: approximately five minutes

✓ Aerobic work: approximately 15 to 20 minutes

✓ Active post-aerobic cool-down: at least five to 10 minutes (or longer if needed for heart-rate recovery)

✓ Final stretching/relaxation: at least five to 10 minutes, longer if time permits

Total-body Workout with Aerobic Work Preceding Strength Work

✓ Warm-up: at least 10 to 15 minutes

✓ Aerobic work: approximately 15 to 20 minutes

✓ Active post-aerobic cool-down: at least five to 10 minutes (or longer if needed for heart-rate recovery)

✓ Brief stretching: approximately two to five minutes

✓ Strength training: approximately 15 minutes*

✓ Final stretching/relaxation: at least five to 10 minutes, longer if time permits

* Intensive strength training should be followed by a few minutes of gentle, active cool-down activity (such as walking or stationary cycling) prior to stretching.

Note: The outlines presented above represent examples of workable exercise formats, but are not intended to cover all viable training options. To keep workout length manageable (approximately JJ159

Table 5.8

Use of Music in Older Adult Movement Classes

Below are several important considerations for incorporating music into group fitness classes:

✓ Music selection should always reflect the unique preferences and physiological needs of a given exercise group.

✓ Remember that the primary purpose of using music is to motivate participants. Do not detract from their exercise experience by being a perfectionist with regard to specific dance steps and precise choreography. In senior aerobics classes, more so than in other adult classes, individual participants may not always move in sync together or even on the correct beat. The instructor should maintain a flexible, fun-oriented attitude.

✓ Older-adult participants tend to prefer lower volume levels than do younger adult participants.

✓ Using instrumental music (as opposed to music that features vocals) may make it easier for some participants to hear the leader's instructions.

✓ Compared to land-based programs, aqua classes call for a slightly slower music tempo since water resistance tends to slow movement. Likewise, constantly trying to move in beat with the music may be less viable during water exercise than during land exercise.

✓ Certain forms of programming (including stretch and relaxation activities) are best conducted without attempting to strictly choreograph the physical movements in compliance with a specific musical beat. In such cases, pleasing music can still be played simply to create an optimal atmosphere. This exception also often applies to chair-seated exercise classes for very frail or disoriented participants.

✓ With practice and experience, accomplished instructors develop an ability to design or adapt appropriate exercise routines using nearly any type of music. However, these general recommended tempo ranges (classified by beats per minute) for land-based senior fitness classes may prove helpful: (1) warm-ups: 100s (or fewer) to 120s; (2) aerobics: 120s to 140s; (3) post-aerobic cool-downs: 100s (or fewer) to 120s; (4) muscle conditioners: 110s to 130s; and (5) stretches: 100s (or fewer).

Chair exercise offers wide training intensity options. An active chair exercise class might include optional standing work using the back of the chair for balance support. It might feature energetic seated aerobic activity involving all of the limbs in broad, synchronized movement patterns. The chair also provides a secure position for the use of resistive exercise accessories such as dumbbells, exercise bands and ankle weights. On the other hand, chair classes can serve extremely disabled participants with poor prognoses who, nonetheless, will benefit from performing limited programs comprised of gentle stretch, posture and breathing exercises.

Following are examples of the types of exercises that can be conducted in a chair-seated class:

Chair Warm-up Techniques

✓ As time permits, include gentle posture and breathing exercises. (See the section on chair-based posture and breathing techniques that follows.)

✓ Perform heel raises (Fig. 5.1).

✓ Perform toe raises.

✓ Circle feet at the ankles.

✓ Alternate turning toes inward and outward (Fig. 5.2).

✓ Alternately curl and then lift the toes.

✓ "Walk" in place.

✓ Perform knee lifts (Fig. 5.3).

✓ Perform knee extensions (optional: combine with arm extensions) (Fig. 5.4).

✓ Move knees together and apart.

✓ Lift shoulders.

✓ Circle shoulders.

✓ Move shoulders forward and backward.

✓ Reach arms forward, upward, out to the sides and down at the sides (Fig. 5.5).

✓ Perform arm circles and sweeps.

✓ Perform elbow and wrist bends (Fig. 5.6).

✓ Open and close hands.

✓ Perform additional hand and finger work (such as moving the fingers apart and together or simulated piano playing).

✓ Perform rocking chair motions.

✓ Perform trunk rotation (Fig. 5.7).

✓ Perform slow, gentle head turns.

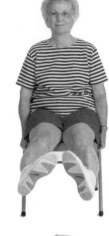
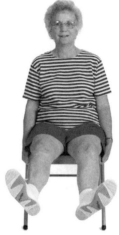

FIGURE 5.2A-B
Toes in/out

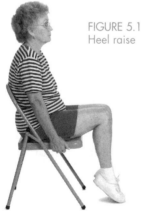

FIGURE 5.1
Heel raise

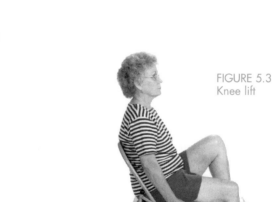

FIGURE 5.3
Knee lift

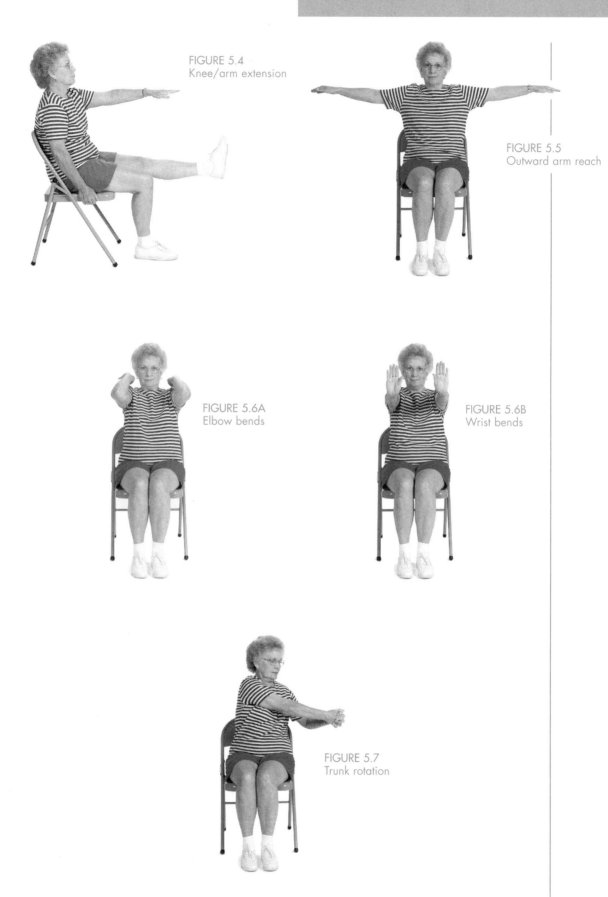

FIGURE 5.4
Knee/arm extension

FIGURE 5.5
Outward arm reach

FIGURE 5.6A
Elbow bends

FIGURE 5.6B
Wrist bends

FIGURE 5.7
Trunk rotation

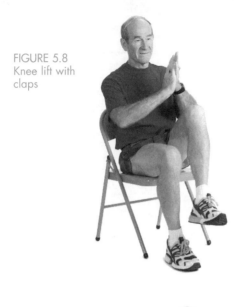

FIGURE 5.8
Knee lift with claps

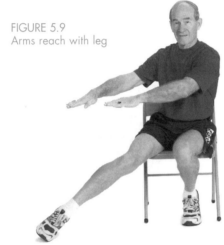

FIGURE 5.9
Arms reach with leg

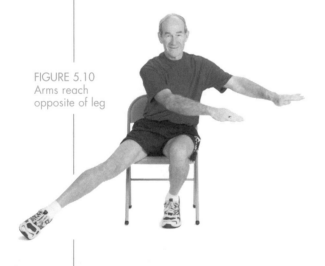

FIGURE 5.10
Arms reach opposite of leg

Chair Aerobic Exercise Techniques

Combine various leg movements with complementary arm movements. Begin the leg movements first, then add the arm motions.

✓ Alternately tap toes to the front.

✓ Alternately tap toes as far as possible out to the sides.

✓ Combine front and side toe taps to form a new leg pattern.

✓ Perform controlled kicks.

✓ Alternate knee lifts with controlled kicks.

✓ Perform cross-over touches to the front.

✓ March in place, bringing knees high (be careful to touch feet to the floor lightly).

✓ Clap hands in sync with leg movements (Fig. 5.8).

✓ Snap fingers in sync with leg movements.

✓ Alternately clap hands and snap fingers in sync with leg movements.

✓ When extending either leg out to the side, reach in the same direction with both arms (Fig. 5.9).

✓ Perform the leg movement in the previous exercise, but reach in the opposite direction with arms (Fig. 5.10).

Chair Post-aerobic Cool-down Techniques

Repeat easy-paced rhythmic movements similar to those used during the warm-up period. Then gently and briefly stretch the upper body, back, hamstrings, quadriceps, calves and shins to prepare the joints and surrounding tissues for strength training. (See stretch section that follows.)

Chair Muscle-strengthening Techniques

Resistance can be incorporated into the following exercises through the use of manual resistance (utilizing one's own hands), gentle pressure against the floor and exercise accessories such as balls, exercise bands and dumbbells. (Suggested means for increasing resistance are listed after each exercise.) A good alternative technique is to have participants progress to wearing ankle weights during leg work and holding them during upper-body work, especially since some participants find them easier to grasp than dumbbells.

✓ Perform upright rows (resistive tubing) if well tolerated. This exercise is not recommended for participants who may be susceptible to shoulder impingement (Fig. 5.11).

✓ Perform chest presses (resistive tubing).

✓ Perform overhead presses (resistive tubing or dumbbells).

✓ Perform overhead pull-downs (resistive tubing).

✓ Perform chin and neck retraction: Without tilting the chin upward, alternately move it back and then release (resisting with palms of hands on back of head).

✓ Perform biceps curls (resistive tubing or dumbbells) (Fig. 5.12).

✓ Perform triceps extensions (resistive tubing or dumbbells) (Fig. 5.13).

✓ Perform rotator cuff conditioning: With upper arms fixed against sides and forearms remaining parallel to the floor, alternately move hands together and then as widely apart as possible (resistive tubing or dumbbells).

✓ Perform scapular retraction: Move shoulders back bringing the shoulder blades close together (dumbbells).

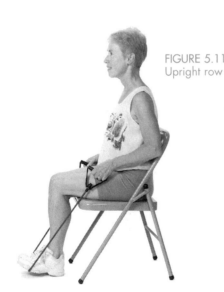
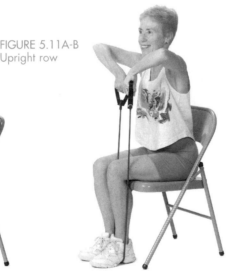

FIGURE 5.11A-B
Upright row

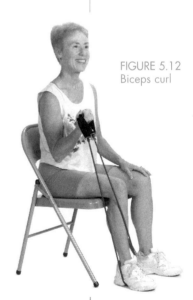

FIGURE 5.12
Biceps curl

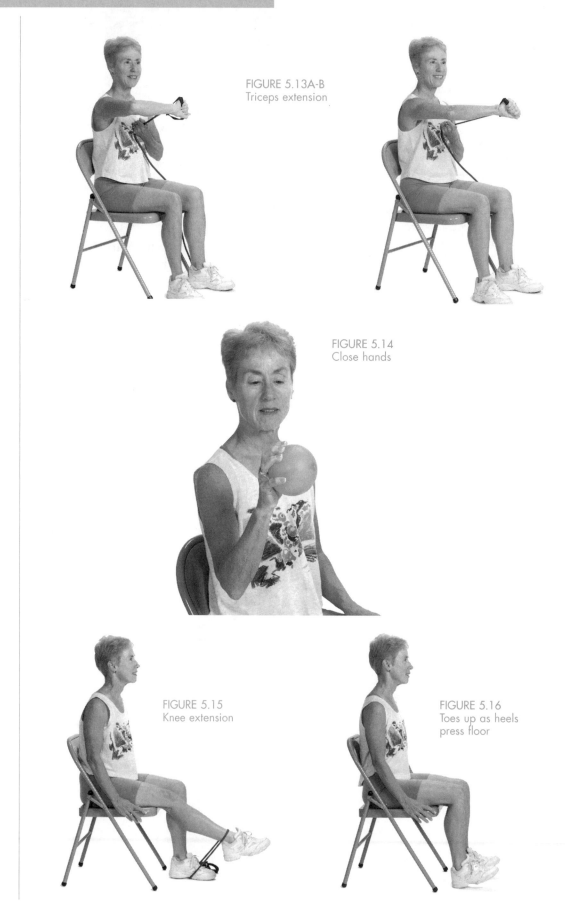

FIGURE 5.13A-B
Triceps extension

FIGURE 5.14
Close hands

FIGURE 5.15
Knee extension

FIGURE 5.16
Toes up as heels
press floor

✓ Perform forearm and wrist turns. For example, simulate turning a door knob (resistive tubing or dumbbells).

✓ Alternately relax and close hands (holding a soft foam ball for resistance) (Fig. 5.14).

✓ Perform hamstring curls with one side of buttocks on chair seat, thereby freeing the opposite leg for movement (resistive tubing).

✓ Perform knee extensions (resistive tubing) (Fig. 5.15).

✓ Perform thigh abduction (resistive tubing) and adduction (large ball placed between knees).

✓ Include plantarflexion and dorsiflexion by performing closed kinetic chain point/flex movements of the feet (pressing floor for resistance) (Fig. 5.16).

Chair Stretching Techniques

✓ Perform ear-toward-shoulder stretches: Lower ear toward shoulder, then return head to upright position (Fig. 5.17).

✓ Perform neck rotation: Turn head toward shoulder (Fig. 5.18).

✓ Perform shoulder/back release: In a slow and controlled manner, move the shoulders in a circular motion upward, back, down, then relax (Fig. 5.19).

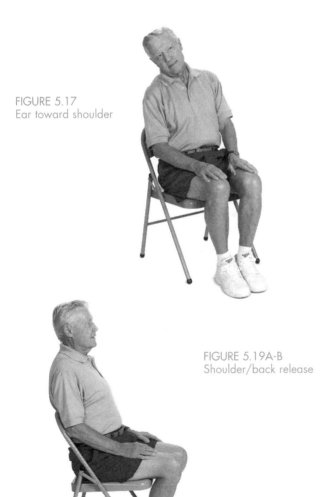

FIGURE 5.17
Ear toward shoulder

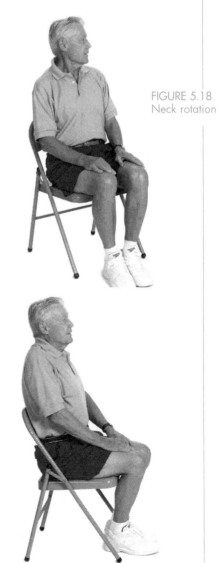

FIGURE 5.18
Neck rotation

FIGURE 5.19A-B
Shoulder/back release

✓ Perform spinal extension/flexion: Begin with both hands placed on the top of the mid-thigh for spinal support, then gently extend and round the back (Fig. 5.20). (Spinal flexion is not recommended for participants with osteoporosis.)

✓ Using "ballet-" styled motions, raise both arms overhead in a high arc. Lower arms in an arc to the lap (Fig. 5.21).

✓ Stretch the trunk: Turn torso toward side, holding onto the same side of chair with both hands.

✓ Stretch the chest and shoulders: With arms bent at the elbows, reach behind the body trying to cross the lumbar spine (Fig. 5.22A). This can help to prepare the participant for another good exercise, the functional stretch: With hands behind the back (one elbow aimed upward and the other downward), bring the fingertips of one hand as close as possible to those of the other (Fig. 5.22B). Since many participants will not be able to touch one hand with the other, emphasize the importance of stretching whether or not hands actually meet.

✓ Perform hip extension: Sitting close to the front edge of the chair (positioned sideways with one side of the body facing the back of the chair, allowing free movement of the opposite hip and leg), reach foot back, angling knee down toward the floor with thigh becoming perpendicular to the floor (Fig. 5.23).

✓ Perform hamstring/gluteal stretch: With hands on thighs, extend leg forward while keeping heel on the floor. Gradually bend forward at the hips (Fig. 5.24).

✓ Stretch inner thighs: Separate knees as far apart as possible.

✓ Stretch outer thighs: Cross one leg over the opposite leg (not recommended following hip replacement surgery until specific medical clearance is granted) (Fig. 5.25).

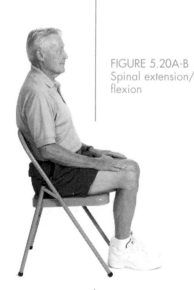

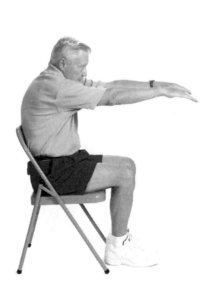

FIGURE 5.20A-B
Spinal extension/flexion

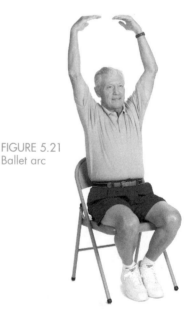

FIGURE 5.21
Ballet arc

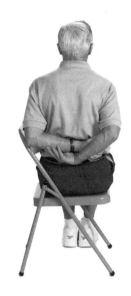
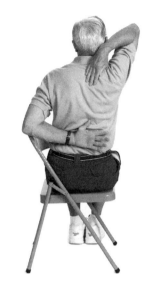

FIGURE 5.22A-B
Arms cross lumbar spine/functional stretch

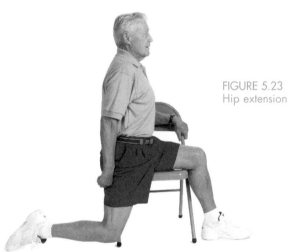

FIGURE 5.23
Hip extension

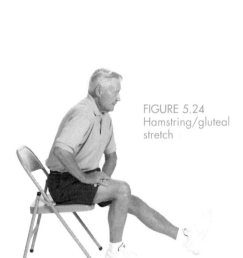

FIGURE 5.24
Hamstring/gluteal stretch

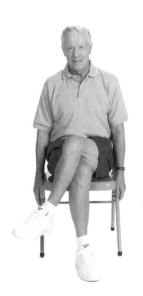

FIGURE 5.25
Outer thigh stretch

✓ Stretch shins/calves with open kinetic chain point/flex: Lift foot (or both feet) and point toes, then slowly pull toes back toward the shin (Fig. 5.26).

Chair Posture and Breathing Techniques

The following exercises also represent enjoyable relaxation activities. They may be incorporated into the warm-up and/or cool-down segments of a class. (Of course, proper breathing instructions, including cautions against breath-holding, are essential during all modes of exercise.)

✓ Achieve neutral spine posture positioning by moving pelvis forward and backward until the most comfortable position is achieved. Then move the ribs and thoracic spine forward and backward until the most comfortable position is achieved. While keeping the chin parallel to the floor (not tilted up or tucked under), move the head forward and back until the most comfortable position is achieved.

✓ Perform weight distribution exercise: With palms up, place hands under the pelvic bones (the bony tips of the ischium). Adjust so that weight feels evenly distributed on both hands.

✓ Conduct posture-awareness exercise: Alternately slouch and then sit up straight, consciously noting the difference between how the two positions feel.

✓ Stabilize the spine: Reach up toward the ceiling with one arm while reaching down toward the floor with the other. Straighten arms as much as possible, trying to reach through the length of the fingertips. Repeat with arm positions reversed.

✓ Perform deep breathing exercise: Take a full breath, then breathe out through pursed lips, allowing the flow of air to make a soft sound as it is pushed out. Expel the last of the air by pretending to blow out a candle. After all possible air has been released, pause for a moment, then repeat.

✓ Inhale normally, but exhale slowly: Breathe in for a count of two, then exhale for a count of four. Breathe in for a count of two, then exhale for a count of six. Breathe in for a count of two, then exhale for a count of eight. Breathe in for a count of two, then exhale for a count of 10.

✓ Perform intercostal breathing exercise: Place hands on the lower rib cage with fingers touching. Inhale deeply so that the rib cage expands and fingers separate. Repeat.

Note: See the aquatic exercise and balance-training sections for activities that may be undertaken while standing and using the back of the chair for balance support.

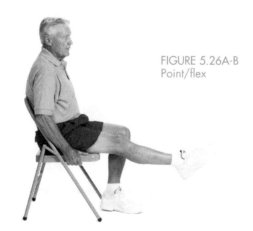
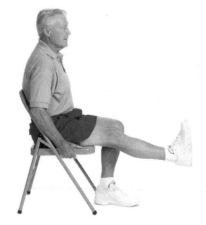

FIGURE 5.26A-B
Point/flex

Low-impact Aerobics Class Techniques

Low-impact aerobic dance is the cardiovascular activity of choice for many older adults. Most classes also incorporate strengthening and flexibility work. Below are specific precautions that should be observed (in addition to all basic safety guidelines) to ensure a safe and enjoyable class:

✓ When conducting a thorough warm-up, pay special attention to warming up the feet and ankles prior to conducting choreographed aerobic dance activities.

✓ Begin with base steps, and always return to a neutral starting position before initiating new patterns.

✓ Use gradual transitions.

✓ Cue clearly and well in advance.

✓ Teach footwork before arm work.

✓ Vary moves to avoid over stressing weight-bearing joints. Always use low-impact choreography.

✓ Balance use of the body (for example, knee lifts with leg curls).

✓ Balance directional changes (for example, front and back with right and left).

✓ Balance moving and stationary patterns.

✓ Avoid quick changes that might compromise balance.

✓ Avoid abrupt or severe turns or twisting that might compromise joints (particularly the knee joint).

✓ Avoid a competitive atmosphere.

✓ Avoid the use of resistance equipment during the aerobics portion of the workout. (Reserve it for the muscle-strengthening segment of the workout.)

Aerobics Class Warm-up Techniques

Refer to the foregoing section on warm-up and cool-down techniques. Also note that most of the warm-up activities listed in the chair-seated section can be adapted to a standing position for use in low-impact aerobics classes.

Aerobics Class Low-impact Techniques

Begin with the leg motions, then add the arm motions.

✓ March: Keeping fists loose, alternately swing each elbow back while marching in place or moving about (Fig. 5.27).

✓ Lift knees: Alternate raising one knee and then the other toward the front as high as feels comfortable, while pushing both arms in various directions (Fig. 5.28).

✓ Perform lift-kicks: Without locking the knees, alternately raise one leg and then the other toward the front while sweeping both arms back and forth across the front (Fig. 5.29).

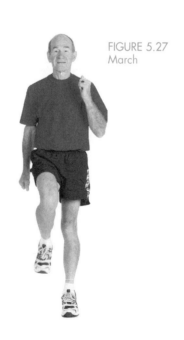

FIGURE 5.27
March

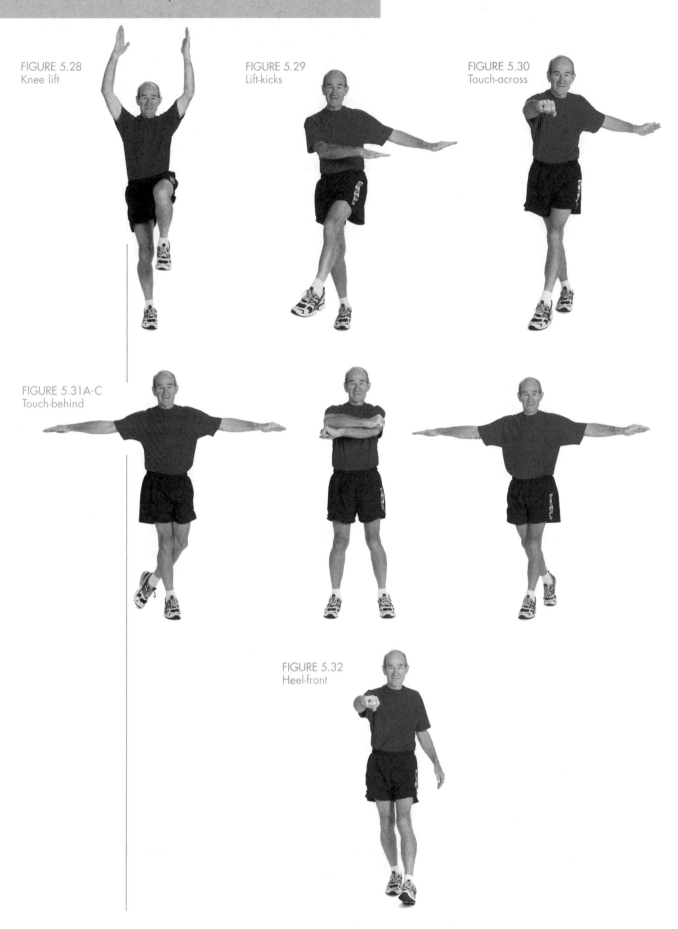

FIGURE 5.28
Knee lift

FIGURE 5.29
Lift-kicks

FIGURE 5.30
Touch-across

FIGURE 5.31A-C
Touch-behind

FIGURE 5.32
Heel-front

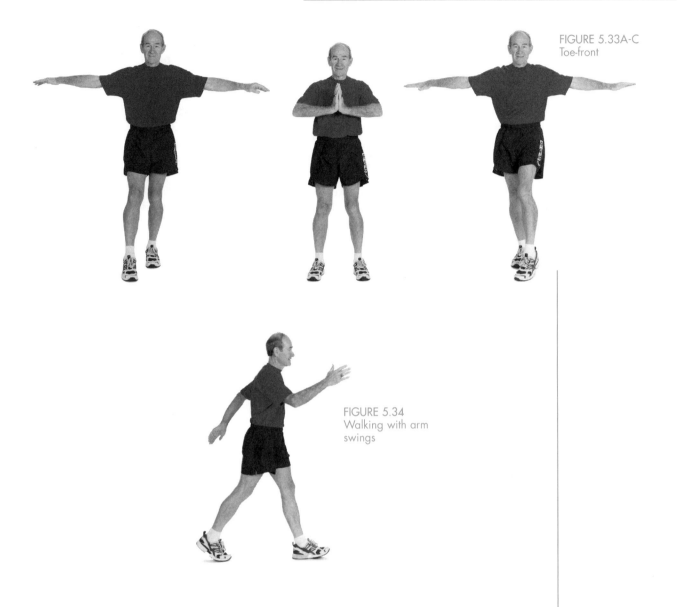

FIGURE 5.33A-C
Toe-front

FIGURE 5.34
Walking with arm
swings

✓ Touch across: Alternately touch the toes of one foot in front of the other foot while performing alternate punches with the arms (Fig. 5.30).

✓ Touch behind: Same movement as above, but touch the toes of one foot behind the other while performing scissor motions with the arms (Fig. 5.31).

✓ Perform heel-fronts (or toe-fronts): Alternate touching one heel (or the toes of one foot) and then the other heel (or toes of the other foot) to the front while reaching forward or clapping with the hands (Figs. 5.32 & 5.33).

✓ Perform toe-outs (or heel-outs): Same as above except touch toes or heels out toward the sides while pushing with the arms or performing side arm raises.

✓ Create combinations: Mix and match the movements described above to develop new patterns and variations.

✓ Perform specific combination #1 (Fig. 5.34): Walk in place, alternately taking slow steps for a specified number of beats, then taking quick steps for a compatible number of beats. Simultaneously perform alternate arm swings to the front and back.

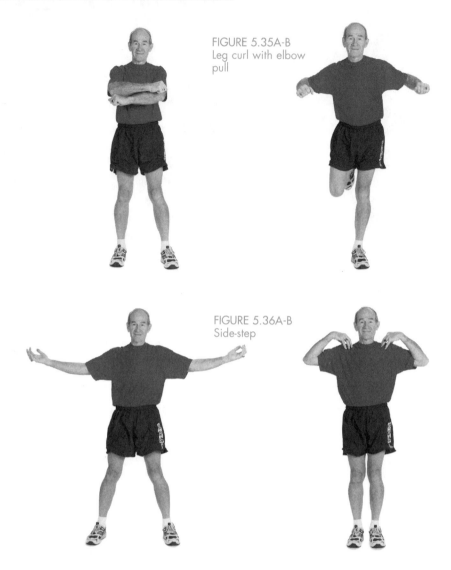

FIGURE 5.35A-B
Leg curl with elbow pull

FIGURE 5.36A-B
Side-step

✓ Perform specific combination #2 (Fig. 5.35): Take 3 steps in place (foot 1, foot 2, foot 1) followed by a leg curl using leg 2; then take 3 steps in place (foot 2, foot 1, foot 2) followed by a leg curl using leg 1. Repeat while holding the arms bent at chest level during the steps and then pulling both elbows back during the curls. For variety, substitute knee lifts for leg curls.

✓ Perform traveling technique #1 (Fig. 5.36): Perform side-stepping by taking several side steps to the right followed by an equal number of side steps to the left (back to starting position). Add any compatible arm movements, such as shoulder touches.

✓ Perform traveling technique #2: Take several steps forward followed by an equal number of steps back (to starting position). Add any compatible arm movements, such as biceps curls. (Persons with balance problems should not step backward; they should step forward in any direction, take several steps in place while turning to face a new direction, then step forward in that direction so they are always facing the direction in which they are moving.)

✓ Perform traveling technique #3: Add variety to side steps or forward-back patterns by performing a low number of knee lifts, small kicks, leg curls, shallow squats or some other special movement while standing in place at each end of the side-stepping or forward-back pattern.

✓ Organize group maneuvers: Achieve interaction through partner or whole-group movements. For example, have couples link arms at the elbows and then switch partners square-dance style, hold hands to form a circle and then use side steps to turn the circle like a wheel, or form a conga line.

✓ Consider creative alternatives: Use the safety guidelines in Table 5.1 to modify line and folk dances, as necessary, to develop senior-appropriate aerobic dance patterns.

Aerobics Class Post-aerobics Cool-down Techniques

Perform easy-paced rhythmic movements similar to those performed during the warm-up period. Then gently and briefly stretch the upper body, back, hamstrings, quadriceps, calves and shins to prepare the joints and surrounding tissues for strength training. (See stretching section that follows.)

Aerobics Class Standing and Floor Exercises for Muscle Strengthening

Note: See the aquatic exercise and balance-training sections for standing exercises that can be performed during aerobics classes by using a ballet bar, the wall or another stable means of balance support. Also, see the chair-seated section for exercise band activities and additional muscle-strengthening exercises that can be adapted to either a floor-seated and/or standing position.

Many older adults can safely benefit by progressing to the use of dumbbells during the following eight shoulder, back, arm and chest exercises:

✓ Perform shoulder lifts and circles (Fig. 5.37).

✓ Perform bent-arm lateral raises (only to a height below shoulder level and if well tolerated) (Fig. 5.38).

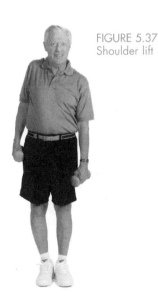

FIGURE 5.37
Shoulder lift

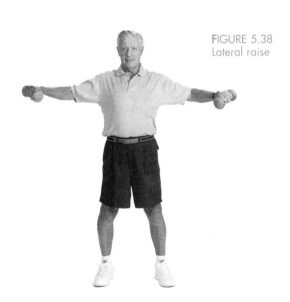

FIGURE 5.38
Lateral raise

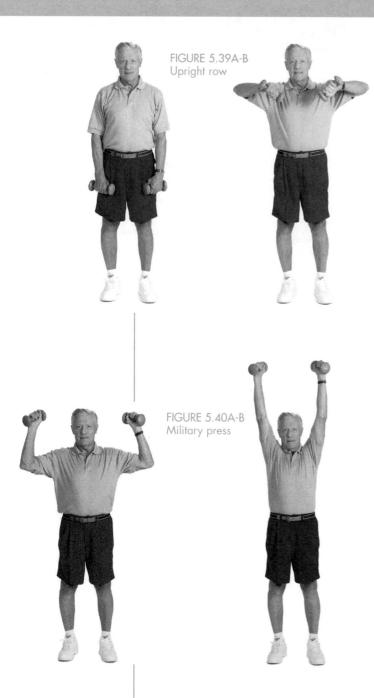

FIGURE 5.39A-B
Upright row

FIGURE 5.40A-B
Military press

✓ Include upright rowing if well tolerated (not recommended for participants who may be susceptible to shoulder impingement) (Fig. 5.39).

✓ Perform military presses (being cautious not to permit excessive vertical loading of the spine, particularly for participants with back problems) (Fig. 5.40).

✓ Perform biceps curls (Fig. 5.41).

✓ Perform triceps extensions (to the back for lighter intensity; higher intensities can be achieved through upward extension) (Fig. 5.42).

✓ Perform supine chest presses (Fig. 5.43).

✓ Perform scapular retraction.

✓ Incorporate chest/back exercise variations: Additional chest and back exercises that do not require the use of weights, bands or other forms of resistive equipment include bent-knee push-ups on the floor, wall push-ups and cat curls on the floor or in a back-supported standing position (Fig. 5.44).

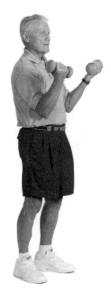

FIGURE 5.41
Biceps curl

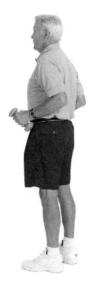
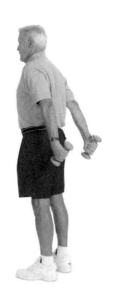

FIGURE 5.42A-B
Beginner's triceps
extension

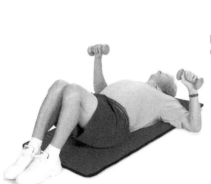
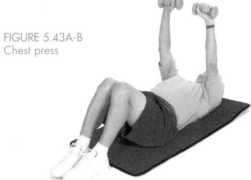

FIGURE 5.43A-B
Chest press

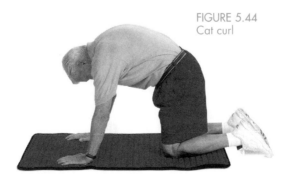

FIGURE 5.44
Cat curl

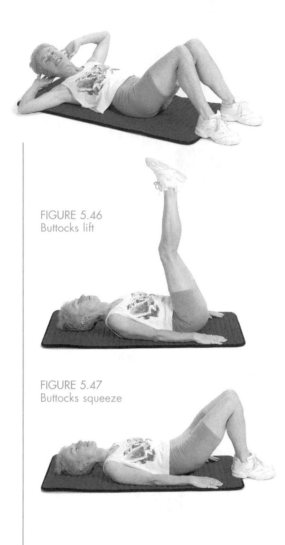

FIGURE 5.45
Diagonal curl-up

FIGURE 5.46
Buttocks lift

FIGURE 5.47
Buttocks squeeze

FIGURE 5.48
Lift

✓ Perform modified vertical and diagonal curl-ups (smoothly rolling the upper body forward to raise it just high enough to clear the shoulder blades off the floor. Take care not to hyperflex the neck.) (Fig. 5.45).

✓ Include lower abdominal exercise: Lie on back with arms at sides, palms on floor and legs held above body. Being careful not to swing or rock the legs, lift buttocks slightly off the floor, then return to starting position (Fig. 5.46). If an easier alternative is needed, perform pelvic tilts: With knees bent and feet on floor, lift buttocks slightly while pressing lower back to floor and contracting the abdominals.

✓ Perform buttocks squeezes: Alternately squeeze and relax the buttocks muscles (Fig. 5.47).

Many older adults can safely benefit by progressing to the use of leg weights during the following five exercises;

✓ Condition back of the thigh: In a prone position, perform small leg lifts. The knee also may be flexed and extended in this position. If needed, a towel or thin pillow may be placed beneath the abdominal/hip area to maintain a neutral spine position (Fig. 5.48).

✓ Condition front of the thigh: Alternately flex and extend the leg forward (Fig. 5.49).

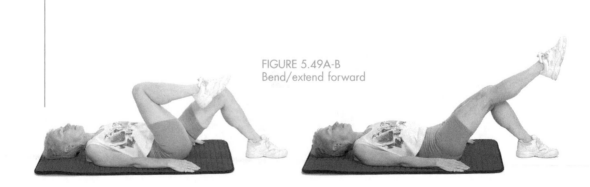

FIGURE 5.49A-B
Bend/extend forward

✓ Condition the inner thigh: Perform lifts with lower leg (not recommended following hip replacement surgery until specific medical clearance is granted) (Fig. 5.50).

✓ Condition the outer thigh: Perform lifts with the upper leg (Fig. 5.51).

✓ Condition shins and calves: Alternately raise heels and then toes (utilizing balance support as necessary) (Fig. 5.52).

Aerobics Class Standing and Floor Exercises for Stretching

Note: Many of the stretches described in chair-seated exercise section can be adapted to either a standing and/or floor-exercise position.

✓ Perform range-of-motion work for the neck: Perform head turns, tilts to the sides (but not back, which may over-compress cervical vertebrae), and nods (Fig. 5.53). Nods should be performed conservatively without pressing the chin toward the chest (which may put excessive pressure on the neck area or over-stretch muscles of the cervical spine area). The safest approach for persons with cervical spinal osteoporosis or arthritis is to avoid nodding exercises.

✓ Perform shoulder stretch: While resting one arm in the bend of the opposite elbow, allow it to stretch gently across the chest (Fig. 5.54).

✓ Perform chest stretch: With fingertips touching shoulders, move elbows back (Fig. 5.55).

FIGURE 5.50
Lower-leg lift

FIGURE 5.51
Upper-leg lift

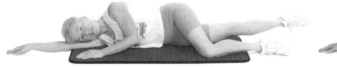

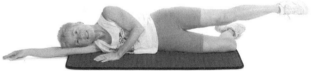

FIGURE 5.52
Heel raise

FIGURE 5.53
Nod

FIGURE 5.54
Shoulder stretch

FIGURE 5.55
Chest stretch

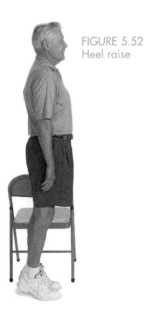

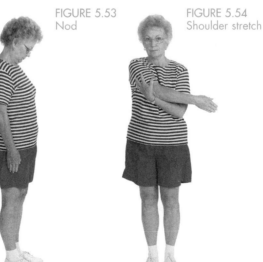

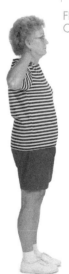

✓ Perform biceps stretch: Extend both arms upward or downward (Fig. 5.56).

✓ Perform triceps stretch: Place hand at back of neck. Grasp the elbow with opposite hand, then pull it gently and slowly toward the back of the head (only so far as feels comfortable) (Fig. 5.57).

✓ Perform midsection and back stretch: With knees bent, reach both arms overhead. Older adults who are able to keep their lower back from arching upward from the floor can maximize this stretch by simultaneously stretching the legs in the opposite direction on the floor (Fig. 5.58).

✓ Perform hamstrings/buttocks stretch: Gently pull legs toward chest (being careful to place hands behind, rather than around, the knees) (Fig. 5.59).

✓ Perform quadriceps stretch: Lying on the stomach, bend leg upward until a pleasant stretch is felt at the front of the thigh. It is easier to relax into an effective stretch if one holds the foot of the bent leg with the hand on the same side of the body; however, trying to do so may exceed arm reach and thereby hyperflex the knee joint. A practical alternative is to loop a towel around the leg to extend the participant's range of motion and

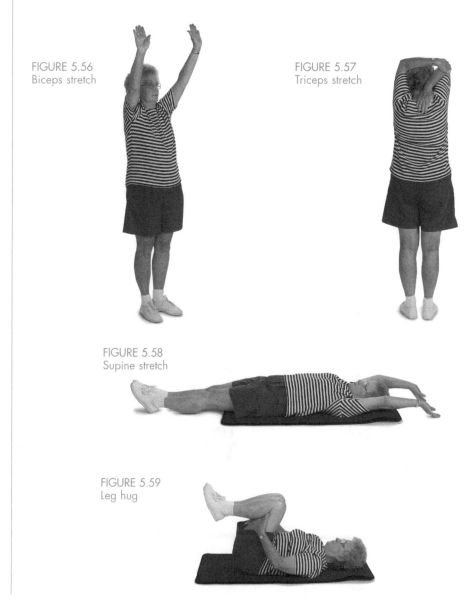

FIGURE 5.56
Biceps stretch

FIGURE 5.57
Triceps stretch

FIGURE 5.58
Supine stretch

FIGURE 5.59
Leg hug

allow the control necessary to ease into an optimally stretched position. The quadriceps may also be stretched in a side-lying position (Fig. 5.60).

✓ Perform inner-thigh stretch: With relaxed knees, separate legs as far apart as feels natural. If this position is un-comfortable, extend one leg at a time slightly toward the side while bending (but not hyperflexing) the opposite knee toward the front. Stretch several parts of the body by placing both hands on the floor in front of you for support while relaxing the upper body slightly forward (Fig. 5.61).

✓ Perform outer-thigh stretch: With one leg bent and crossed over the other, press the knee gently toward the floor with the opposite hand. Press conservatively so that only a pleasant stretch, not a pulling sensation, is felt along the outer thigh. Variation #1: If the hip is allowed to cross over, the lower back will be stretched (Fig. 5.62). Variation #2: Increase the stretch for the hip area by gently pulling the bent, crossed leg to-ward the chest (a supine piriformis stretch). This exercise is not recom-mended following hip replacement surgery until specific medical clearance is granted.

✓ Perform wall calf stretch: With both hands on the wall, lean forward keeping both heels on or near the floor. (Avoid sinking into a swayback posture and hyperextending the knees or elbows.) Note: The shins and calves can be stretched in a floor-exercise position by slowly performing and holding open kinetic chain point/flex movements with the feet (Fig. 5.63). Likewise, ankle range of motion can be promoted in various positions, including on the floor, by performing slow open kinetic chain circular movements of the feet.

Note: If desired, incorporate activities from the following balance training and relax-ation sections or from the posture/breathing portion of the preceding chair-seated section into the final cool-down stretch period.

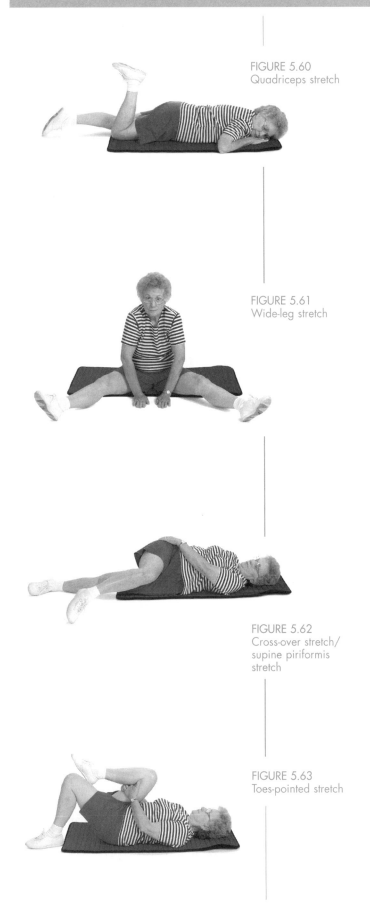

FIGURE 5.60
Quadriceps stretch

FIGURE 5.61
Wide-leg stretch

FIGURE 5.62
Cross-over stretch/
supine piriformis
stretch

FIGURE 5.63
Toes-pointed stretch

Aquatic Programming Techniques

While the same principles and safety guidelines that govern other forms of exercise pertain to water exercise as well, several special considerations also apply:

✓ Complete lifeguard certification or have a qualified lifeguard present during classes.

✓ Remove unnecessary obstacles from the pool deck and sweep it free of slippery water spots. Regularly inspect the condition of the pool, its railings, ladders and shower areas.

✓ Never touch electronic sound equipment while wet or when standing on a damp surface.

✓ A flat pool floor surface is preferable to one that slopes. Wearing non-skid aqua shoes can help prevent slipping and may offer extra cushioning for the joints.

✓ In outdoor pools, the skin should be protected by sun screen. Sunglasses can safeguard the eyes, and tinted goggles are available for those whose eyes are sensitive to pool chemicals.

✓ A water temperature of 87° to 88° F works well for most older adult group class designs.

✓ Instructors who teach on the pool deck (instead of in the water) can see, and be seen better by, participants. A good view of the instructor is important because pool areas often have poor acoustics and are made noisy by splashing water. Also, some participants who normally use hearing aids will not wear them during water classes.

✓ It is generally considered more viable to monitor intensity level during water aerobics by RPE rather than by heart-rate counting (M. Sanders, personal communication, July 31, 1997).

✓ Accessories made for in-pool use such as water bells, paddles, webbed gloves and ankle cuffs can be incorporated to increase intensity and/or to help participants float during selected activities.

✓ Exercises that require holding onto the wall in order to keep both feet above the pool floor can strain the upper body. Seek alternative positions in which the participant floats or keeps at least one foot in contact with the pool floor.

✓ As in all older adult training, avoid needlessly hyperextending the joints. During standing leg lifts, for example, remind participants not to support their body weight on a hyperextended knee.

✓ As in all older adult training, emphasize neutral spine techniques; one swimming pool exercise that can aggravate a bad back is flutter kicks with unsafe hyperextension of the back.

✓ Because water's buoyancy takes most of the jolt out of exercise, many older adults who cannot safely jog, jump or kick on land can successfully do so in the pool. Still, all senior adults should monitor the response of joint tissue to movements that involve hopping or bouncing—even in water. If joint stress or pain is experienced, substitute lower-impact activities.

Aquatic Warm-up Techniques

Refer to the foregoing section on warm-up and cool-down techniques. Also note that most of the warm-up activities listed in the chair-seated section can be adapted to a standing position for use in aquatic exercise classes. The water walking activities described below can be used during the warm-up or the aerobic segment, depending upon participant performance level. The warm-up period is an excellent time to practice personal safety skills such as skulling for balance and recovering in-balance posture (with both feet securely beneath the body).

Aquatic Aerobic-training Techniques

The aerobics segment of the workout can consist of water walking, choreographed aerobic movements, or some combination of both. A general rule is to alternate periods of more strenuous work (such as energetic knee lifts) that last up to approximately one minute with periods of less strenuous work (such as jogging in place) lasting approximately half a minute to control intensity. It may be desirable to conduct more than one class to accommodate the training needs of participants at different fitness levels.

Note: Some dance steps from the aerobics section can be adapted for use in the water. Coordinate arm and leg movement for optimal balance and stabilization.

Water walking activities and variations:

✓ Walk in the center of the pool or while touching the pool wall for balance support.

✓ Walk in place, forward, back, sideways, diagonally, in a circular pattern or from one side of the pool to the other and back.

✓ Walk on the entire foot, on the toes, on the heels, with toes aimed straight ahead, turned out or turned in.

✓ Walk with legs in a naturally extended position, or with knees slightly bent.

✓ Walk in a natural forward-moving fashion, as though walking a line, with high knee lifts, knee lifts out toward the sides, extra long strides, or with controlled kicking motions.

✓ Rather than walking, jog, run or leap through the water.

✓ Along with lower body movements, perform various arm motions such as the crawl stroke, the back stroke, the breast stroke, the dog paddle, punches, pushes and sweeps.

✓ Choose a depth at which the participant can control their body's buoyancy in the water while maintaining an effective speed of movement.

Other aquatic aerobic moves:

✓ Hop on both feet (touching down as lightly as possible without hyperextending the knees upon landing) (Fig. 5.64).

✓ Alternately hop on one foot, then the other (without exceeding four consecutive hops per foot for joint safety).

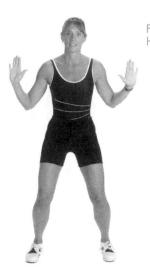
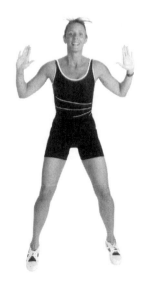

FIGURE 5.64A-B
Hop

✓ Perform chorus-line-style kicks (Fig. 5.65).

✓ Perform jumping jacks with different types of arm movements and jumping jack variations, such as alternately extending one leg and then the other upon landing (Fig. 5.66).

✓ Perform alternate high knee lifts to the front and/or sides.

✓ Perform frog jumps: With knees to the sides, pull both feet up as high as possible under the body, then return to standing posture (Fig. 5.67).

✓ Perform bobbing movements: Extend left leg back while right knee remains bent to the front, then quickly reverse leg positions. Continue alternating, being careful to keep the front knee behind the front toes and the back knee relaxed upon landing (Fig. 5.68).

✓ Practice skilled movements: If participants can swim and tread water, consider including lap swimming or treading in shallow water so that it is possible to stand occasionally as necessary.

Aquatic Post-Aerobics Cool-Down Techniques

Perform easy-paced rhythmic movements similar to those performed during the warm-up period. In general, broad sweeping movements are better than short, reduced-range movements. Gently and briefly stretch the upper body, back, hamstrings, quadriceps, calves and shins in order to prepare the joints and surrounding tissues for strength training. (See stretch section that follows.) Keep active enough for participants to stay warm, for example, by alternating stretch exercises with lower body movements such as walking or easy-paced jogging.

Aquatic Muscle-strengthening Techniques

For upper body work, participants should assume a stance in which they feel stable and in balance. Many older adults feel most secure with feet a comfortable distance apart and one foot in front of the other.

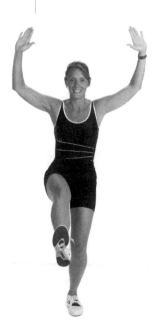

FIGURE 5.65
Kick

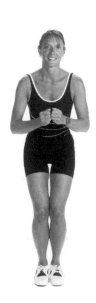

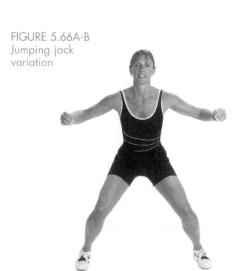

FIGURE 5.66A-B
Jumping jack
variation

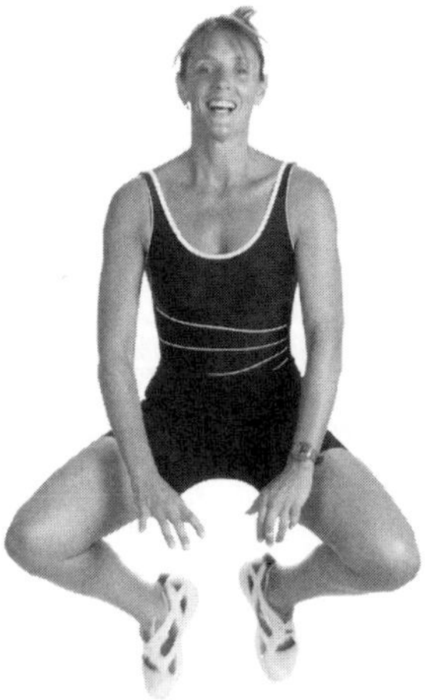

FIGURE 5.67
Frog jump

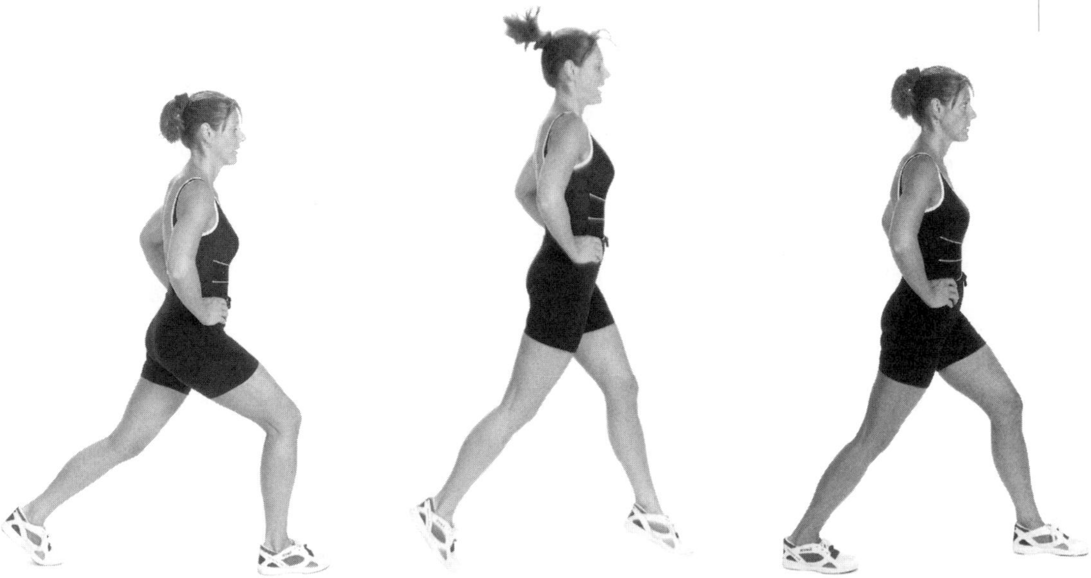

FIGURE 5.68A-C
Bob

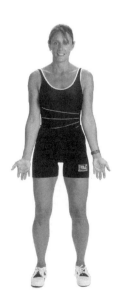
FIGURE 5.69A-B
Biceps/triceps
strengthener

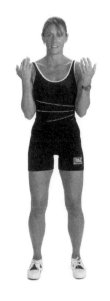

✓ Perform biceps/triceps strengthener: Alternately flex and extend the elbow against water resistance. Start with arms at sides, palms up; with upper arms remaining against the body and elbows remaining pointed downward, bend the elbows and raise the hands toward the shoulders; while hands are at shoulder level, turn the palms forward and straighten the elbows, pressing hands down to starting position. Then turn palms up and repeat (Fig. 5.69).

✓ Incorporate shoulder strengtheners: Perform arm lifts in various directions (e.g., toward the front or back).

✓ Include chest/upper-back strengthener #1: In a scissor-like manner, cross arms in front of the body, open out to the sides, then cross behind the back. Continue alternating. To add resistance, turn palms as necessary to ensure maximum water displacement throughout the movements (Fig. 5.70).

✓ Include chest/upper-back strengthener #2: Start with arms out to the sides, palms forward; move arms together in front of the body; return to starting position, consciously squeezing shoulder blades together as arms move back (Fig. 5.71).

✓ Include upper-body multi-muscle strengthener: Perform pool wall push-ups.

✓ Perform trunk stabilizer: Start with both arms extended together in front of the chest with palms touching; pull arms toward one side and then the other, allowing the torso to turn gently from side to side with the arms (Fig. 5.72).

✓ Perform abdominal/back strengthener: Simply undertake walking activities in relatively shallow water (e.g., waist deep) while focusing intently on maintaining optimal posture.

FIGURE 5.70A-C
Arm scissors

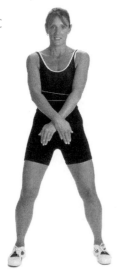
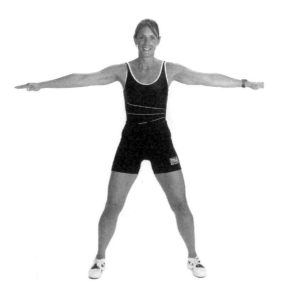
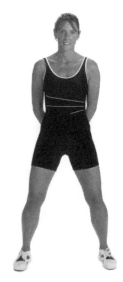

The following exercises which use the pool wall as a ballet bar are suitable for beginners. Progression may involve performing increasingly more challenging variations of the work: (1) without touching the wall, (2) while holding foam dumbbells, (3) while wearing webbed gloves, (4) while traveling, and (5) while keeping hands out of the water.

✓ Perform front-of-thigh strengthener: Using the pool wall as a ballet barre (touch the wall for balance, but do not lean on it), perform bent-knee leg lifts to the front as well as knee flexion/extension to the front (Fig. 5.73).

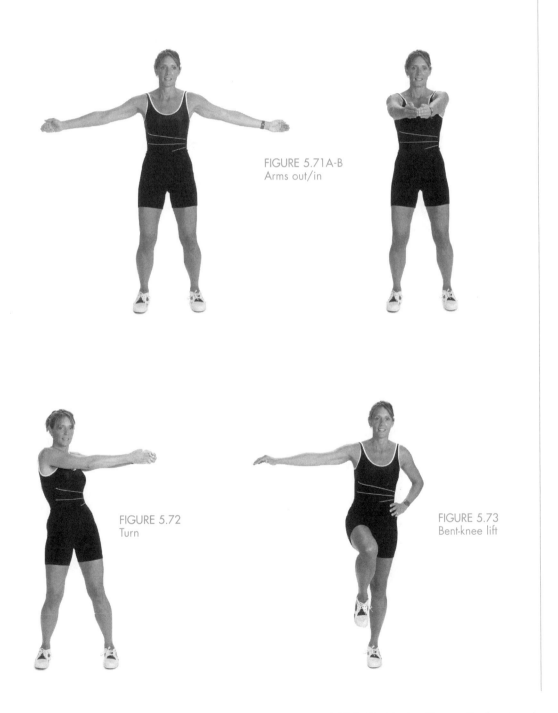

FIGURE 5.71A-B
Arms out/in

FIGURE 5.72
Turn

FIGURE 5.73
Bent-knee lift

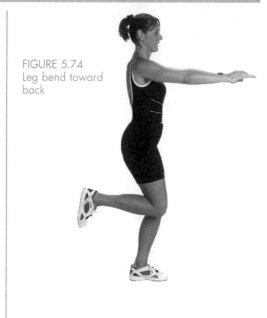

FIGURE 5.74
Leg bend toward
back

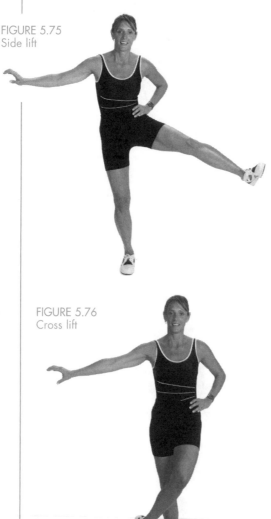

FIGURE 5.75
Side lift

FIGURE 5.76
Cross lift

✓ Perform back of thigh strengthener: Using the pool wall as a ballet bar, perform backward leg lifts by bending at the knee to raise the foot up toward the buttocks (Fig. 5.74).

✓ Perform outer thigh strengthener: Using the pool wall as a ballet bar, perform leg lifts to the side (Fig. 5.75).

✓ Perform inner thigh strengthener: Using the pool wall as a ballet bar, perform leg lifts in front of the opposite leg (not recommended following hip replacement surgery until specific medical clearance is granted) (Fig. 5.76).

✓ Perform shin/calf strengthener: Using the pool wall as a ballet bar, alternately raise the toes, then the heels (Fig. 5.77).

Note: Some of the strengthening and stretching exercises from the aerobics class section and the chair-seated section also can be adapted for use in the water.

Aquatic Stretching Techniques

During flexibility work, keep active enough to stay warm, for example, by alternating stretch exercises with lower-body movements such as walking or easy-paced jogging.

✓ Stretch the neck: Perform head turns, tilts and/or nods.

✓ Stretch biceps: Fully extend both arms, either overhead or down in the water.

✓ Stretch triceps: Place one hand on the other at the nape of the neck. Slowly slide hands down until elbows point up (Fig. 5.78). To vary this exercise, slide the hand down the forearm to meet the other hand at the nape of the neck. Reach both hands down the back.

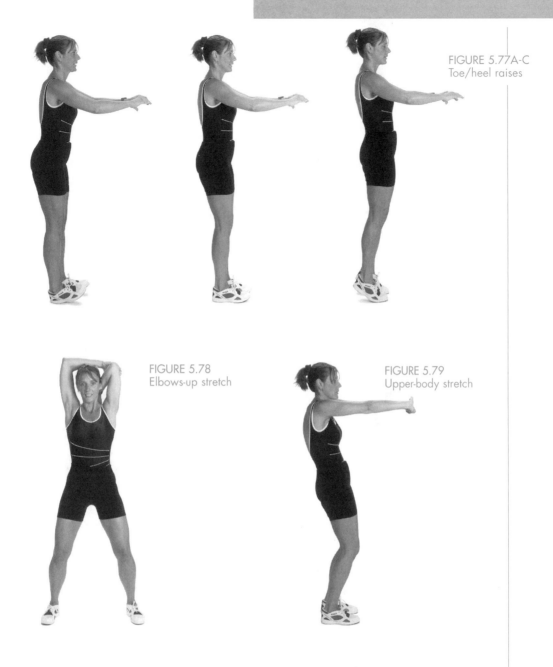

FIGURE 5.77A-C
Toe/heel raises

FIGURE 5.78
Elbows-up stretch

FIGURE 5.79
Upper-body stretch

✓ Stretch upper back/shoulders: Interlace fingers, palms facing forward, and stretch both arms to the front. Then relax arms down by the sides and perform slow shoulder circles, first backward, then forward (Fig. 5.79).

✓ Perform back/posture stretch: Press the back to the pool wall while standing as tall as possible. Keeping the rib cage elevated, press the shoulders back and down while reaching toward the floor with the fingers.

✓ Stretch chest: With hands on hips, gently press shoulders back.

✓ Stretch trunk: Stand with side to the pool wall and feet together at arm's length from the edge. Touch wall with the arm closest to the wall (extended but relaxed). First pull hips away from the wall while reaching in overhead with the outside arm. Then, with the rib cage elevated, reach up toward midline. Finally, pull hips toward wall while reaching down and out with the same arm. Repeat facing opposite direction (Fig. 5.80).

✓ Stretch quadriceps: With knee aimed downward, raise foot to the back. To better relax into the stretch, grasp the ankle with the hand that is on the same side of the body. If grasping the ankle is difficult, try grasping the heel. Do not hyperextend the back or touch the heel to the buttock (which hyperflexes the knee).

✓ Perform hamstring/gluteal stretch: With hands placed behind (not around)

the knee, first perform a gentle leg hug, then extend the leg at the knee until a pleasant stretch is felt along the back of the thigh. (If balance support is needed, stand with back to pool wall.) (Fig. 5.81).

✓ Stretch outer thigh: Cross one leg in front of the other until a pleasant stretch is felt along the outer thigh (not recommended following hip replacement surgery until specific medical clearance is granted) (Fig. 5.82).

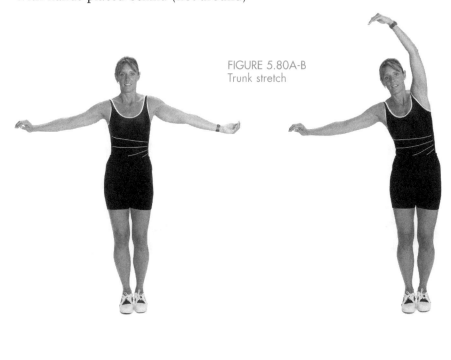

FIGURE 5.80A-B
Trunk stretch

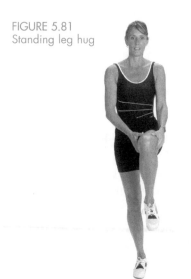

FIGURE 5.81
Standing leg hug

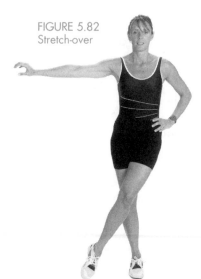

FIGURE 5.82
Stretch-over

✓ Stretch inner thigh: Facing the wall with feet apart, shift hips to the side, causing one leg to bend as the other stretches. Repeat in opposite direction (Fig. 5.83).

✓ Stretch shin: Using the pool wall as a ballet bar, point toes (Fig. 5.84).

✓ Stretch calf: Using the pool wall as a ballet bar, flex foot (Fig. 5.85).

Relaxation Class Techniques

Relaxation activities can be incorporated into any type of fitness programming format, whether it be a seated exercise class, a low-impact aerobics class, aquatics, fitness walking or personal training. It is best included at the end of the exercise session. On the other hand, you can conduct classes fully devoted to relaxation. However it should be made clear to participants that relaxation programming alone does not constitute a complete, well-balanced fitness regimen and that they will need to augment the class with other forms of exercise.

It is important to create an atmosphere conducive to relaxation programming. If practicable, dim the lighting somewhat and block out sounds from outside the immediate area. Use smooth, calming music such as symphonic selections. Or try audio tapes featuring captured nature sounds such as wind, rain, muted thunder and rolling waves. Probably the most essential key to success will be the instructor's voice and demeanor. Speak slowly, quietly and soothingly. Avoid sudden or unnecessary movements, and any tendency to rush. Do not allow any hurried sense to arise during relaxation activity.

Elements of the following relaxation techniques can be used singly during the final cool-down/stretch segment of

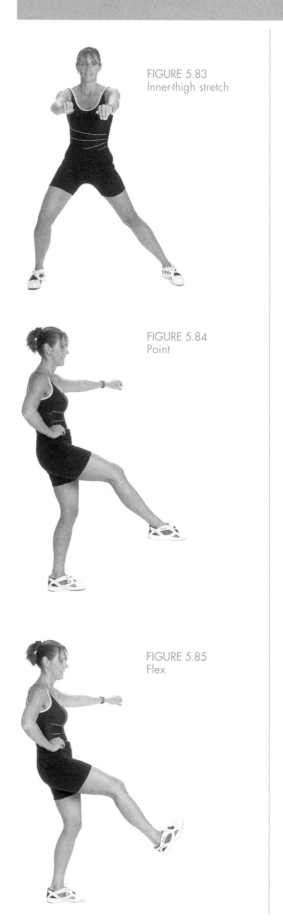

FIGURE 5.83
Inner-thigh stretch

FIGURE 5.84
Point

FIGURE 5.85
Flex

an exercise session or in combination within the context of a more comprehensive relaxation program.

✓ In aquatic settings, the water itself can be a relaxation programming device. Water has a pleasurable stroking effect as it surrounds, massages and laps against the body. Setting aside several minutes for complete personal relaxation at the end of aquatics class is a good way to capitalize on the water's natural properties. Allow participants a peaceful, unstructured period to simply float or lounge in the water, perform breathing exercises or undertake their choice of quiet activity.

✓ Stretching and gentle range-of-motion activities can be especially relaxing. Refer to all of the stretches described in this chapter as a resource. Also, yoga-styled classes are renowned for their ability to relax and de-stress participants.

✓ Soft, tactile or aromatic accessories can be utilized to promote reposeful, enjoyable sensations. For example, sensory-based activities might include luxuriously applying hand lotion or handling a plush, feathery or fur-like fabric or object.

✓ Relaxation methods can involve techniques as simple as including poignant lines of poetry, brief inspirational quotations, thoughts for the day, simple stress-management tips or positive self-talk activities during the final moments of a class.

✓ Relaxing self-massage can be performed in a number of ways. For example, have participants lightly sweep their fingers through their hair, gently rub their skeletal muscles and softly caress their skin. Do not massage the neck (except quite lightly at the very back) since this can interrupt blood flow.

Note: Gentle posture and breathing exercises can be a valuable addition to relaxation programming. For seven good activity

examples, refer to the posture/breathing segment of the chair-seated technique section on page 156.

Below are some additional specific techniques:

✓ Perform gentle posture activity #1: In a chair-seated position, sit back on the hips. With both hands placed on top of the thighs to provide support for the spine, lean forward and back several times (bending from the hips, not from the waist), then lean from side to side several times. Continue adjusting position until upper-body weight feels evenly distributed.

✓ Perform gentle posture activity #2: In a chair or floor-seated position, interlace fingers with palms facing forward. Raise arms overhead. Hold for one or two long breaths, then relax and lower arms. Repeat.

✓ Perform gentle posture activity #3: In a chair or floor-seated position, place hands behind head. Move elbows back while pulling the chin in. Keeping chin parallel to the floor (not tipped upward or tucked down), gently move head back into the hands. Slowly turn head to the right, then to the left. Repeat.

✓ Perform breathing exercise #1: In a chair or floor-seated position, inhale deeply, attempting to fill the bottom of the lungs. Note the pressure of the breath on the chest and abdomen as the air rises toward the top of the lungs. Exhale, releasing air from the top of the lungs first, then from the bottom. Repeat.

✓ Perform breathing exercise #2: In a chair or floor-seated position, with both hands placed on the top of the thighs to support the spine, lean forward from the hips while exhaling as fully as possible. While returning to an upright position, attempt to refill the lungs with air by sniffing "like a dog" five or six times. Repeat.

✓ Perform breathing exercise #3: In a chair or floor-seated position, pull both elbows backward while inhaling deeply. With back slightly arched, hold breath for a count of five. Push air out by gently contracting the abdominal muscles. Repeat several times.

✓ Conduct simple, progressive muscular-relaxation activities. For example, while lying flat on the back with eyes closed, begin with the head and move down to the toes. Mentally focus on one muscle group at a time, first noting any tightness present, then inhaling fully. While slowly exhaling, envision the tension flowing out of the muscles and completely out of the body along with the breath. When the procedure is completed, rest quietly for a few minutes before getting up.

✓ Another method of progressive relaxation: While seated or lying down, focus on each muscle group, working down from head to toe. First, tense the muscle for approximately two seconds, noticing how this feels; second, release the tension, again noticing how this feels; third, pause and reflect upon the difference between the two sensations before moving on to the next muscle group.

✓ Incorporate pleasurable mental imagery to help participants relax. Developing effective graphic description skills may take practice. Have participants recline and close their eyes. Remember to speak in a slow, soothing manner. Note that in the following example, reference to the senses of touch, sight, hearing and smell are all woven into the imaginary scenario: *Feel yourself gliding easily on your back down a broad, lazy stream in the forest. The stream is so clear and pure that if you turn your head only slightly, you can discern through its shear, emerald waters thousands of tiny polished stones scattered like precious jewels on the stream bed. Without a care in the world, you can feel the sunlight warming your skin and the cool water caressing your arms, your legs, your back and your sides as you float peacefully along the shimmering stream. Feel the gentle tickle of a light breeze playfully teasing at your face. Hear the echo of a bird's song as it drifts down from the thick, green foliage of the surrounding forest. Breathe deeply the fresh, sweet fragrance of the velvety moss and ferns that grace the water's edge; breathe deeply the heavy perfume of exotic flora blooming recklessly along the stream's verdant banks. Just float and dream ... float and dream ... as the forest's natural treasures lull you into a peaceful reverie.*

Balance/Coordination Training Techniques

As in other forms of senior fitness programming, balance training's possibilities are limited only by the fitness professional's skills and creativity. Certain types of sports, such as tennis, promote balance skills in people who can safely enjoy them. Even equine therapy is used by qualified professionals to increase the balance and coordination of disabled participants. Various types of ball play, such as tossing, catching, batting and aiming, can be implemented for coordination and balance purposes. (In chair-seated classes, a partially inflated beach ball works particularly well.) Tai Chi is another excellent means of balance/coordination training.

Performing balance work in a swimming pool can lessen participants' fear of falling. Land-based balance activities can be undertaken while facing a wall, ballet bar or the back of a sturdy chair for support. In some land-based exercise groups, participants are capable of providing one another with mutual support during balance training by working as partners or standing in a circle while holding hands.

Many factors can contribute to imbalance. Therefore, various interventions ranging from disease management, medication adjustments, glasses/eyesight correction and many forms of physical activity training may be appropriate in addressing such problems. Participating in a complete, well-balanced fitness program is probably the most critical factor for maintaining and preserving adequate balance. However, there are certain techniques that can be employed that are specifically designed to recruit and sharpen balance mechanisms. Several of these are listed below.

The following exercises should be done in a standing position with balance support available. Safety should be the primary consideration during balance training and in all other forms of older adult physical training.

✓ Stand with feet approximately shoulder width apart and extend arms out slightly forward and lower than the shoulders. Lift both heels off the floor and try to hold the position for 10 seconds.

✓ Standing with feet side by side, hold arms in the same position as described in the previous exercise. Place one foot on the inside of the opposing ankle and try to hold the position for 10 seconds. Repeat with hands behind the back (Fig. 5.86).

✓ Perform a one-legged stand with one foot raised to the back (the non-weight-bearing knee flexed 90°). Try to maintain the position for a minimum of three seconds. The long-term goal is to decrease the need for balance support and to hold the position for 10 seconds. However, as necessary, allow the hands to contact the provided support apparatus.

✓ Perform the same exercise as above, but raise one foot to the front (the non-weight-bearing knee flexed and lifted approximately as high as the hip) (Fig. 5.87).

✓ Transfer body weight onto one foot and lift the other slightly off the floor. Reverse, then continue alternating weight-shift/foot-lift movements from one side to the other.

✓ With the knee straight but not hyperextended, execute single (relatively small) leg raises to the front, then the back. Continue alternating front to back (Fig. 5.88).

FIGURE 5.86
Foot on opposite ankle

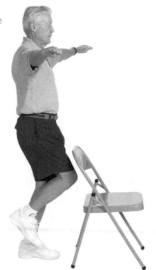

FIGURE 5.87
Knee flexed to front

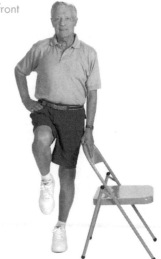

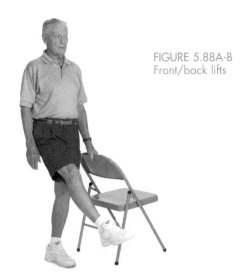
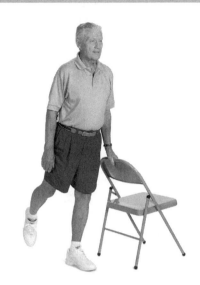

FIGURE 5.88A-B
Front/back lifts

✓ Assume the same position as in the previous exercise, but alternate small leg raises to the side with raises toward the inside (slightly past the central axis of the body if no hip range restrictions exist).

✓ Design a balance-training program based on recent scientific research findings, such as those derived from the following sensory-training project (Woollacott, 1995). In that study, older adults were instructed to stand under eight different conditions, 10 seconds in each stance, five times apiece, 10 different times per day, for 10 days. The eight conditions involved standing:

1. on a firm surface, eyes open, head neutral

2. on a firm surface, eyes closed, head neutral

3. on a firm surface, eyes open, head tilted back

4. on a firm surface, eyes closed, head tilted back

5. on a foam surface, eyes open, head neutral

6. on a foam surface, eyes closed, head neutral

7. on a foam surface, eyes open, head tilted back

8. on a foam surface, eyes closed, head tilted back

Balance mechanisms were called upon as progressively more difficult conditions provided lesser degrees of accurate sensory feedback from the environment. At the end of the trial, sway had decreased under all conditions, significantly so in the most difficult positions. Improvement occurred in the ability to stand on one leg, a skill that transfers into routine tasks of daily living.

The investigators' experience suggests that this training should be ongoing. When the study ended, the subjects' performance levels declined after four weeks without training. Incorporating the activity into year-round older adult fitness programs may enhance clients' balance and lower their risk for falls.

For obvious reasons, great care must be taken to ensure client safety during such activity. Whereas tilting the head backward and standing with one's eyes closed both are highly questionable activities in other older adult exercise situations, both are integral to this balance training design. Therefore, this type of training is not for everyone. It requires cautious screening as well as a carefully controlled, well-supervised environment that reflects the provision that all potential safety issues have been anticipated, analyzed and addressed in advance to ensure the individual client's continuing physical safety. Examples of risk-reducing precautions include: 1) omitting the backward head tilt for participants with neck problems; 2) reminding all participants to open their eyes and/or utilize balance support as frequently as they deem personally necessary.

Fitness Walking Techniques

The general guidelines for aerobic training as outlined earlier in this chapter should be applied to older adult fitness walking programs. In addition to those basic criteria, several special considerations also should be kept in mind when planning walking activities for older participants:

✓ Environmental considerations: Do not conduct outdoor walking activities when the temperature exceeds 85° F or the humidity exceeds approximately 60 percent. Do not walk in extreme cold (which can cause lung discomfort or hypothermia), when wind chill is immoderate, when air pollution levels pose a risk or when lightning threatens. Have an indoor alternative ready for bad weather days. Avoid walking on dangerous surfaces such as those with holes, obstructions or icy patches, and broken sidewalks.

✓ Apparel and accessories: Make certain that participants are wearing comfortable, supportive walking shoes and clothing appropriate to existing weather conditions. Layered clothing can be removed as the body warms or added if the weather grows cooler. Protect the eyes and skin with sunglasses, visors and sunscreen. Have drinking water available and consume it liberally, especially in hot weather. If possible, walk during daylight hours. If it is necessary to walk after sundown, wear reflective attire. (Individuals should carry identification; those who are not members of a group should walk with a friend whenever possible.)

✓ Warming up and cooling down: Avoid the common mistake of conducting walking-only warm-up and cool-down periods before and after fitness walking sessions. While it is effective to begin with slow walking and progressively increase the pace to limber up and gradually increase circulation, additional warm-up activities should be included to provide a complete warm-up period as described earlier in this chapter. A structured, total-body warm-up may help participants lift their feet slightly higher or swing the arms and legs with greater ease, which can help prevent tripping and add pleasure to the walking experience. Likewise, gradually reducing one's pace toward the end of a walking session is an excellent cool-down component. Walking also should be followed by stretching to foster joint range of motion and to discourage unnecessary soreness or cramping.

✓ Ensuring an effective aerobic workout: A watch and inexpensive pedometer are useful for tracking time and distance. To maintain an adequate aerobic-intensity level, however, it also is important to rate perceived exertion and/ or periodically monitor heart rate. Energy expenditure can be increased by increasing duration or frequency. Speed also may be increased within safe and sensible limits. (Approximately 3 mph is a good goal for most participants.) Persons who do not have problems related to balance, the lower back or the knees can increase intensity by walking on a variable terrain surface including gradual inclines. The use of weights during fitness walking for older adults is controversial. Ankle weights should not be used because they can overstress the back, hips and knees. Wrist weights that are no heavier than 1 pound apiece may be used safely by some individuals; however, they may overstress the back, neck, shoulders and elbows in others. In general, the most prudent approach is to reserve the use of weights for strength-training sessions.

✓ Walking technique: With each step, the heel should touch the ground just before the ball of the foot followed by the toes, effecting a heel-to-toe rolling action. Maintain good posture with relatively loose shoulders and low arms. When the arms are carried too high, unnecessary neck and shoulder tension can result. Allow the arms to swing naturally at sides. Work toward preserving or increasing stride length, as needed.

✓ Special program-planning consideration #1: It is good to vary outdoor walking routes when possible, using local features such as beaches, mountains, parks, wooden walkways, long fishing piers, well-maintained outdoor stairways with railings, bridges, scenic parks and neighborhoods, and interesting historical districts. Only crime-safe walking routes that are free of dangerous traffic conditions should be taken. Regarding any route chosen, advance provisions (such as carrying a cellular telephone), that enable the instructor to summon emergency assistance promptly, if needed, must be in place.

✓ Special program-planning consideration #2: Team teaching works well for outdoor groups with members at different fitness levels. While one instructor sets a pace for the fast walkers (and can lead them on a longer route which eventually circles back to rejoin the other participants), another instructor stays with the slower walkers.

✓ Special program-planning consideration #3: Although indoor walking programs may lack the variety, stimulation and fresh-air qualities of outdoor programs, they do have certain advantages. These include temperature and climate control, no exposure to ultraviolet rays, smooth, unobstructed walking surfaces, and ready access to rest benches, water fountains, rest rooms and telephones. Music can be conveniently incorporated, if desired. Various walking patterns (such as large figure eights and criss-cross routes) may be combined with lap walking for variety.

Personal-training Techniques

Personal trainers are in a special position that allows them to utilize any techniques from previous sections that they deem beneficial. In addition, they can supervise extremely effective forms of training that are best conducted on a one-to-one basis, such as individualized functional-fitness training and strength-machine work.

Note: In personal training milieus, the treadmill and stationary cycle are convenient means for gradually increasing circulation during the warm-up phase and for conducting aerobic training.

Functional-fitness Training

Functional fitness, which defines the parameters of one's ability to perform basic activities of daily living, should influence the practical objectives of older-adult exercise programming. Ideally, fitness specialists seek to train elderly clients for optimal functional performance.

Functional fitness relates to an individual's physical independence in terms of:

✓ Mobility (e.g., standing and walking)

✓ Self-care (e.g., bathing, grooming, and toileting)

✓ Exerting adequate control over one's living environment (e.g., driving and shopping, preparing meals and performing household maintenance tasks)

✓ Preserving specific physical abilities needed for pursuits that enhance quality of life (e.g., entertaining grandchildren, volunteering, gardening, playing golf and traveling)

Through effective functional-fitness training, older adults may be able to avoid, postpone, reduce or reverse declines in physical-performance level. When the training succeeds in decreasing an individual's risk for falling, its value is incalculable.

Personal trainers are in an excellent position to help clients maintain and improve their functional-fitness level. As a general guideline, functional-fitness training should simulate selected real-life tasks. In choosing exercises, consider the day-to-day activities each individual client needs to perform successfully. Specific functional exercises should be undertaken within the broader context of a complete, well-balanced training program. Below are several especially effective functional-fitness training techniques:

✓ Perform gentle neck rotation.

✓ Perform upper-body exercises involving the arms, hands and trunk in lifting, reaching, turning, pulling and pushing.

✓ Simulate everyday stair-climbing tasks by stepping up and stepping down on a low platform (with balance support available).

✓ Perform sit-to-stand activity (moving from a chair-seated position to a standing posture and vice versa).

✓ Perform squats (observing the safety cautions provided below in the resistance-exercise section).

✓ Perform additional lower-extremity strengtheners (such as heel raises).

✓ Perform balance-training activity.

✓ Perform walking activity.

Strength Training

Personal training provides the most efficient means for ensuring that an adequate strength-training intensity is achieved. Remember, the personal trainer is free to use any of the techniques shown in this chapter, adapting them as appropriate to a participant's personal training program.

In intensive strength-training programs, it is a good practice to work larger muscle groups first. For example, the machine and free-weight routines provided below start with the legs, then move to the torso, arms and midsection. Ideally, opposing muscle groups should be worked in succession. Foam pads, foot supports and seat belts can be used to correct alignment problems and ensure stable positioning.

Listed below are resistance-machine exercises for a basic strength-training program and the primary muscles and muscle groups worked:

✓ Leg extension: quadriceps

✓ Leg curl: hamstrings

✓ Leg press: hamstrings, gluteals and quadriceps

✓ Chest cross: pectoralis major and anterior deltoid

✓ Chest press: pectoralis major, anterior deltoid and triceps

✓ Pullover: latissimus dorsi and teres major

✓ Lateral raise: deltoids

✓ Biceps curl: biceps

✓ Triceps extension: triceps

✓ Low-back strengthener: erector spinae

✓ Abdominal curl: rectus abdominus

You also may wish to utilize machinery to focus on the forearms, inner and outer thighs, calves and shins.

Some trainers successfully enlist strength machines that engage the sternocleidomastoids, upper trapezius and levator scapulae through neck flexion, extension, and lateral flexion. The extension phase may be omitted if any tendency toward hyperextension poses a risk to the participant. Other trainers express concern regarding the potential risks of prescribing neck exercises that utilize extrinsic resistance for populations in which pre-existing cervical vertebrae damage is common. Reliable advice can be obtained by consulting the participant's personal physician.

The practice of free-weight training requires extra safety awareness and particularly close supervision for the purpose of spotting. The following free-weight exercises can be implemented cautiously to train most of the major muscle groups:

✓ Squats: hamstrings, gluteals and quadriceps. (Do not lower buttocks below knee level; this exercise is more safely performed with dumbbells than with a barbell.)

✓ Bench press: pectoralis major, anterior deltoid and triceps. (This exercise is more safely performed with dumbbells than with a barbell.)

✓ Bent-over row (single-arm pulls with back supported by placing opposite hand and knee on well-padded bench): latissimus dorsi, teres major and biceps

✓ Alternate arm overhead press using dumbbells: deltoids and triceps

✓ Biceps curls with both arms together using dumbbells: biceps

✓ Triceps extension using dumbbells (single arm extensions with back supported by placing opposite hand and knee on well-padded bench): triceps

✓ Curl-ups (floor exercise holding single plate on chest for resistance): rectus abdominus. (Engage the obliques with diagonal curl-ups.)

Note: For illustrations of these strength-training exercises, see the *ACE Personal Trainer Manual* (2nd Ed).

Conclusion

There is no single best method of training older adults. The best approach is the one that meets the participant's goals and needs *and* that they will perform consistently. Developing an effective, balanced, well-tolerated program that enhances quality of life is a realistic goal. All of the methods described in this chapter are viable, depending upon the individual to be trained. The professional's challenge, as well as the key to success for all involved, is determining and implementing the most appropriate training method or methods for each participant.

References

American College of Sports Medicine. (1995). *Guidelines for Exercise Testing and Prescription* (5th ed). Baltimore: Williams & Wilkins.

American College of Sports Medicine. (1990). *Guidelines for Exercise Testing and Prescription* (4th ed). Philadelphia: Lea and Febiger.

Borg, G.A.V. (1982). Psychophysical bases of perceived exertion. *Medicine & Science in Sports & Exercise,* 14, 377-381.

Charette, S.L., McEvoy, L., Pyka, G., Snow-Hart, C., Guido, D., Wiswell, R.A. & Marcus, R. (1991). *Muscle Hypertrophy Response to Resistance Training in Older Women.* Palo Alto, Calif.: American Physiological Society.

DeBusk, R.F., Stenestrand, U., Sheehan, M. & Haskell, W.L. (1990). Training effects of long versus short bouts of exercise in healthy subjects. *American Journal of Cardiology,* 65, 1010-1013.

Ettinger, W., Jr., Mitchell, B. & Blair, S. (1996). *Fitness After Fifty: Never Too Late to Start.* St. Louis: Beverly Cracom.

Fiatarone, M.A., Marks, E.C., Ryan, N.D., Meredith, C.N., Lipsits, L.A. & Evans, W.J. (1990). High-intensity strength training in nonagenarians. *Journal of the American Medical Association,* 263, 3029-3034.

Fiatarone, M.A., O'Neill, E.F., Ryan, N.O., Clements, K.M., Solares, G.R., Nelson, M.E., Roberts, S.B., Kehayias, J.J., Lipsits, L.A. & Evans, W.J. (1994). Exercise training and nutritional supplementation for physical frailty in very elderly people. *New England Journal of Medicine,* 330, 1769-1775.

Fletcher, G.F., Balady, G., Froelicher, V.F., Hartley, L.H., Haskell, W.L. & Pollock, M.L. (1995). Exercise standards: A statement for healthcare professionals from the American Heart Association. *Circulation,* 91, 580-615.

Frontera, W.R., Meredith, C.N., O'Reilly, K.P., Knuttgen, H.G. & Evans, W.J. (1988). *Strength Conditioning in Older Men: Skeletal Muscle Hypertrophy and Improved Function.* Palo Alto, Calif.: American Physiological Society.

Gersten, J.W. (1991). Effect of exercise on muscle function decline with aging. *Western Journal of Medicine,* 154, 579-582.

Gladwin, L.A. (1996). Stretching: A valuable component of functional mobility training in the elderly. *Activities, Adaptation & Aging,* 20, 3, 37-47.

Hyatt, G. (1996). Strength training for the aging adult. *Activities, Adaptation & Aging,* 20, 3, 27-36.

Paffenbarger, R.S., Hyde, R.T., Wing, A.L. & Hsieh, C.C. (1986). Physical activity, all-cause mortality, and longevity of college alumni. *New England Journal of Medicine,* 314, 605-613.

Pate, R.R., Pratt, M., Blair, S.N., Haskell, W.L., Macera, C.A., Bouchard, C., Buchner, D., Ettinger, W., Heath, G.W., King, A.L., Kriska, A., Leon, A.S., Marcus, B.H., Morris, J., Paffenbarger, R.S., Patrick, K., Pollock, M.L., Rippe, J.M., Sallis, J. & Wilmore, J.H. (1995). Physical activity and public health: A recommendation from the Centers for Disease Control and Prevention and the American College of Sports Medicine. *Journal of the American Medical Association,* 273, 402-407.

Pollock, M.L., Carroll, J., Graves, J.E., Leggett, S.H., Braith, R.W., Limacher, M. & Hagberg, J.M. (1991). Injuries and adherence to walk/jog and resistance training programs in the elderly. *Medicine & Science in Sports & Exercise,* 23, 1194-1200.

Pollock, M.L., Graves, J.E., Swart, D.L. & Lowenthal, D.T. (1994). Exercise training and prescription for the elderly. *Southern Medical Journal,* 87, 5, S88-S95.

Pollock, M.L., & Wilmore, J.H. (1990). *Exercise in Health and Disease* (2nd ed). Philadelphia: Saunders.

Spirduso, W.W. (1995). *Physical Dimensions of Aging.* Champaign, Ill.: Human Kinetics.

Swart, D.L., Pollock, M.L. & Brechue, W.F. (1996). Aerobic exercise for older participants. *Activities, Adaptation & Aging,* 20, 3, 9-25.

U.S. Department of Health and Human Services. (1996). *Physical Activity and Health: A Report of the Surgeon General.* Washington, D.C.: U.S. Government Printing Office.

Westcott, W.L. (1995). *Strength Fitness: Physiological Principles and Training Techniques* (4th ed). Dubuque, Iowa: William C. Brown.

Woollacott, M. (October 6, 1995). Changes in balance control in the older adult: Effects of balance training programs. (Lecture given at International Conference on Aging and Physical Activity; available on audio tape from Human Kinetics, P.O. Box 5076, Champaign, Ill. 61825).

Recommended Reading

American Senior Fitness Association. (1996). *Long Term Care Fitness Leader Training Manual.* (2nd ed.) New Smyrna Beach, Fla: SFA.*

American Senior Fitness Association. (1996). *Senior Fitness Instructor Training Manual.* (2nd ed.) New Smyrna Beach, Fla: SFA.*

American Senior Fitness Association. (1996). *Senior Personal Trainer Training Manual.* (2nd ed.) New Smyrna Beach, Fla: SFA.*

American Senior Fitness Association. (Quarterly periodical). *The Senior Fitness Bulletin.* New Smyrna Beach, Fla: SFA.*

Clark, J. (Ed.). (1996). *Exercise Programming for Older Adults.* New York: Haworth Press.

Clark, J. (1993). *Full Life Fitness: A Complete Exercise Program for Mature Adults.* Champaign, Ill.: Human Kinetics.

Clark, J. (1988). *Seniorcise: A Simple Guide to Fitness for the Elderly and Disabled.* Sarasota, Fla.: Pineapple Press.

Coven, E. (1992). *Seniorobics: The Fitness Guide for People 55+.* Jericho, NY: FitWise Programs, Inc.**

Ettinger, W., Jr., Mitchell, B. & Blair, S. (1996). *Fitness After Fifty: Never Too Late to Start.* St. Louis: Beverly Cracom.

Evans, W. & Rosenberg, I.H. (1991). *Biomarkers: The 10 Keys to Prolonging Vitality.* New York: Fireside (Simon & Schuster).

Sanders, M., Rippee, N. (1993) (videos). Speedo Aquatic Fitness System: Instructor Training Course Videos. ****

Sova, R. (1995). *Water Fitness After 40.* Champaign, Ill.: Human Kinetics.

Van Norman, K.A. (1995). *Exercise Programming for Older Adults.* Champaign, Ill.: Human Kinetics.

Westcott, W.L. & Baechle, T.R. (1998). *Strength Training Past 50.* Champaign, Ill.: Human Kinetics.

Westcott, W.L. (1996). *Building Strength and Stamina: New Nautilus Training for Total Fitness.* Champaign, Ill.: Human Kinetics/Nautilus International.

Wilson, M.A. (1996). *Caregiver's Guide to Exercise.* Spokane, Wash.: Sit and Be Fit.***

*Available from the American Senior Fitness Association, P.O. Box 2575, New Smyrna Beach, Fla. 32170 (telephone 800-243-1478, fax 904-427-0613).

**Available from FitWise Programs, P.O. Box 759, Jericho, NY 11753 (telephone 516-822-6306).

***Available from Sit and Be Fit, P.O. Box 8033, Spokane, Wash. 99203-0033 (telephone 509-448-9438).

****Available from Speedo International, Ltd., 5591 E. Rainbow Ridge Ct., Reno, NV 89523 (telephone 800-999-4332).

Acknowledgments

The author wishes to extend special thanks to Wayne Westcott, Ph.D., Laura Gladwin, M.S., Mary Sanders, M.S., Mary Ann Wilson, R.N., Ellen Coven, M.A., Kay Van Norman, M.S. and Gwen Hyatt, M.S., whose publications provided many of the specific exercise techniques described in this chapter.

EXERCISE

programming
and leadership

Kay Van Norman

Kay Van Norman, M.S., physical education and health, has taught at Montana State University for 16 years and is the director of Young at Heart, an exercise program that involves more than 200 senior citizens in water aerobics, arthritis water exercise, chair exercise, low-impact aerobics and strength training. She is an authority on exercise programming for seniors, giving presentations on older adult fitness and wellness at numerous national and international conferences each year.

Van Norman is the author of Exercise Programming for Older Adults, and served as the national chair of the Council on Aging and Adult Development within the American Alliance for Health, Physical Education, Recreation and Dance from 1995 to 1997. During this time she authored the CAAD's nationally published position statement on the need for quality exercise programming and instruction for older adults. She also is a member of the National Coalition to Develop Standards for Senior Exercise Specialists and a reviewer for the newly developed Rickli/Jones Functional Fitness Tests for Independent Older Adults.

Safe and effective programming for older adults requires integrating knowledge of their special needs with appropriate assessment procedures and exercise techniques, giving special attention to program implementation, as well as marketability. This chapter facilitates this integration of concepts by first providing specific strategies for determining current levels of function, identifying and prioritizing specific needs at each functional level, and then identifying programming that effectively meets these needs without exposing participants to unnecessary risks. This integration requires one to carefully form a bridge between the current research on physical activity and aging and exercise programming. This bridge can be built with function-based programming that reflects the practical application of proven concepts (Figure 6.1).

In addition, this chapter provides strategies for applying exercise principles in a way that meets the special needs of seniors, and outlines methods for developing programs to attract seniors from various levels of functional ability. Finally, strategies for the recruitment and motivation of seniors are addressed, along with low-cost equipment options for increasing exercise effectiveness and enjoyment.

Determining the Levels of Function

The range of functional ability within the older adult population can be categorized into five different levels. Spirduso (1995), in her book *Physical Dimensions of Aging,* identifies these levels as: Physically Dependent, Physically Frail, Physically Independent, Physically Fit and Physically Elite. Her definitions provide a useful framework for identifying the functional abilities and needs of each level.

Physically Dependent

The physically dependent older adult cannot execute some or all of the Basic Activities of Daily Living (BADL), including self-dressing, bathing, transferring, using the toilet, feeding and walking. These individuals are dependent on others for food and for basic functions of living.

Physically Frail

Physically frail seniors can perform BADL, but cannot perform some or all of the activities necessary to live independently. This is generally due to a debilitating disease or condition that physically challenges them on a daily basis.

Physically Independent

The physically independent older adult lives independently, usually without debilitating symptoms of major chronic diseases, but has low health and fitness reserves. For many such individuals, a brief illness or injury can mean a rapid loss of physical function and, thus, a loss of independence. Even after recovery from the initial illness or injury, their loss of function results in physical frailty.

Physically Fit

The physically fit senior exercises at least twice per week for their health, enjoyment and well-being, or works regularly at a physically demanding job or hobby. Their health and fitness reserves put them at low risk for falling into the physically frail category.

Physically Elite

The physically elite older adult trains on an almost daily basis to compete in sport tournaments, work in a physically demanding job or participate in recreational activities.

FIGURE 6.1

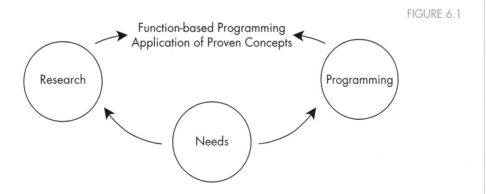

Function-based Programming
Application of Proven Concepts

Research

Programming

Needs

Identifying & Addressing Needs

Pre-screening and physical assessments help you determine each individual's level of physical function. Pre-screening includes inquiring about medical background, medications and pre-existing health conditions.

Refer to Chapter 4 for specific pre-screening and physical assessment strategies. Also, you may refer to Table 6.1 (Spirduso, 1995) for a list of commonly used tests of physical function. Using the appropriate physical assessments will help you identify the client's current level of functional ability and any physical deficits that must be addressed.

Chapter 4 also provides strategies for assessing psychological responses to exercise, including expectations and goals. The psychological aspect of assessment is a critical, but often overlooked, component of developing programming that addresses needs, as well as personal objectives related to exercise participation.

Using both physical and psychological assessments will help you identify the most immediate needs for each individual or group, and allow you to prioritize program goals. For example, whereas aerobic conditioning is very beneficial for older adults, it is of little or no use to someone within the first two levels of functional ability who are struggling to perform BADL. This is where the concept of "movement that matters" becomes useful, i.e., prioritizing and addressing the most immediate physical and psychological needs. Chapter 4 makes reference to this same concept by stating that "assessments should be relevant to the individual's needs and objectives."

Physically Dependent

Movement that helps physically dependent older adults maintain or improve their physical function for basic self-care is important to this group. They need the strength, range of motion, balance and coordination necessary for self-feeding, bathing, dressing, going to the bathroom, transferring and walking. Concentrate on activities to improve finger and hand strength and agility, arm strength, shoulder and hip range of motion, leg strength (especially in the quadriceps and ankle flexors), ankle strength and range of motion, and foot and toe mobility.

Identifying Needs

To provide programming that addresses BADL, it is important to understand the specific physical function necessary for each of the activities. The following outline will help you determine these necessary functions:

Self-toileting requires enough strength and range of motion in the legs and hips to go from a standing to seated and seated to standing position. In the case of a wheelchair-bound individual, it requires upper-body strength for transferring from the chair to the toilet and back. Self-toileting also requires enough strength and range of motion in the hands and arms to remove and replace clothing.

✓ R.O.M. - in the hips, knees, ankles, shoulders and wrists

✓ STRENGTH - in the legs, hips, arms and hands

Self-bathing requires strength and range of motion in the hips and legs to get in and out of the tub. It also requires enough strength and range of motion in the hands and arms to remove and replace clothing and wash all areas of the body.

✓ R.O.M. - in the hips, knees, ankles, shoulders and wrists

✓ STRENGTH - in the legs, hips, arms and hands

Successful self-transferring requires strength and range of motion in the

Table 6.1

Performance Tests of Physical Function in Old and Oldest-Old Adults

Category	Example Tests	Sources
Physically elite	VO$_2$max; modified Balke treadmill	ACSM, 1991
	Bruce treadmill protocol	Bruce, Cooper, et al., 1973
	Resistance strength tests; dynamometry	McArdle, Katch, & Katch, 1991
	Routine flexibility and agility tests	
Physically fit	VO$_2$max, as above	ACSM, 1991
	Resistance strength tests; dynamometry	McArdle, Katch, & Katch, 1991
	Fitness tests:	
	jumping, hand strength, flexion	Kimura et al., 1990
	balance, agility, power, flexibility	Kuo, 1990
	jumping, side-step, flexion, reaction time	Tahara et al., 1990
Physically independent	Tests of low-level physical function	
	AAHPERD field test	Osness, 1987
	Advanced activities of daily living (AADL)	Reuben etal., 1990
Physically frail	Instrumental activities of daily living (IADL)	Lawton & Brody, 1969
	Hierarchical ADL-IADL	Kempen & Suurmeijer, 1990
	GERI-AIMS	Hughes et al., 1991
	Tinetti's mobility assessment	Wolfson, Whipple, Amerman, & Tobin, 1990
	Physical performance test (PPT)	Reuben & Siu, 1990
	Physical impairment scale	Jette, Branch, & Berlin, 1990
Physically dependent	Basic activities of daily living (BADL)	Katz et.al., 1963
	Physical Disability Index (PDI)	Gerety et al., 1993
	Mobility Functioning in Nursing Home Residents	Schelle et al., in press
	Physical Performance and Mobility Exam	Lemsky et al., 1991
	Barthel Index	Mahoney & Barthel, 1965
	Tests of hand function	Jebsen et al., 1969
	Williams board test	Williams & Hornberger, 1984
	Get-Up-and-Go test	Mathias, Nayak, & Isaacs, 1986
	Timed Up-and-Go screening test	Podsiadlo & Richardson, 1989

Spirduso, Waneen (1995). Physical Dimensions of Aging. Human Kinetics.

legs, and balance to sit on, and stand up from, a chair, or transfer to or from a bed. In the case of wheelchair-bound individuals, it requires enough strength in the upper body to transfer from the chair to a bed and from a bed to the chair.

✓ R.O.M. - in the ankles, knees and hips

✓ STRENGTH - in the legs, hips and arms (to aid in rising)

✓ BALANCE - enough to accomplish transfers without falling

Walking requires strength and range of motion in the lower body and enough balance to get from one place to another without falling. Walking with an assistive device also requires strength in the upper body to effectively use the device.

✓ R.O.M. - in the ankles, hips and knees

✓ STRENGTH - in ankles, hips and legs. There is a secondary concern for strength in the upper back to help maintain posture, proper alignment and balance. If an assistive device is being used, additional upper-body strength is necessary.

✓ BALANCE - to transfer weight from one foot to the next, sustain a one-footed stance, and maintain an appropriate stride length and normal gait

✓ CONFIDENCE - in their ability to walk without falling

When choosing exercises to improve performance of BADL, ask yourself three questions:

1) Does this exercise address an immediate need?

2) Will it help improve function?

3) Is there a safer alternative?

When determining programming for individuals in the dependent category with multiple physical impairments, it is always important to weigh the benefits of an exercise against its possible risks. Sometimes a measured amount of risk is acceptable if the benefits are significant. For example, it is extremely important for an individual to maintain the ability to self-toilet. Quadriceps strength plays a large role in this aspect of self care and personal independence. Knee extensions against resistance can significantly improve quadriceps strength but, for some individuals, may also cause discomfort in the knee joint. If modifications do not alleviate the discomfort, but the discomfort is temporary and manageable, the benefits of maintaining enough quadriceps strength for self-toileting are likely to outweigh the risks. Refer to Table 6.2 for programming appropriate for physically dependent older adults.

Table 6.2

Programming for the Physically Dependent

✓ chair-based exercises that specifically address each of the BADL

✓ one-on-one water-based exercise (water walking, range of motion and strength work)

✓ resistance exercise for the upper and lower body

✓ individualized "home-based" exercises

✓ breathing and relaxation

✓ hand function exercise

Physically Frail

Physically frail seniors need exercise that helps them maintain or improve their ability to perform BADL and Instrumental Activities of Daily Living (IADL). IADL are more complex physical abilities such as preparing meals, housecleaning, shopping and mobility in and out of the home. Exercise programming will focus on muscular strength, endurance, flexibility, joint range of motion, balance and coordination.

Identifying Needs

Leg strength significantly contributes to improved balance and the ability to recover from near falls. It also helps clients regain or maintain a normal gait pattern, which includes ankle flexion with heel strike, a full stride length and appropriate gait speed. Programming that focuses on strengthening the upper back and stabilizing the shoulder blades in a neutral position (instead of rounded forward), will help improve posture. For example, encouraging clients to routinely perform scapular retraction (i.e., pulling the shoulder blades together in

Table 6.3

Programming for the Physically Frail

✓ chair-based exercises that specifically address the basic and instrumental activities of daily living

✓ one-on-one water-based exercise (water walking, range of motion and strength work)

✓ resistance exercise to improve upper- and lower-body strength

✓ breathing and relaxation

✓ chair exercise and chair-assisted exercise that practice balance and coordination

✓ group water-based programming that addresses strength, range of motion, balance and coordination

✓ individualized "home-based" exercise

back) throughout the day can help improve posture. Improved posture in turn promotes better balance and gait.

Additional areas to address include foot mobility and agility, which also impact balance and gait. This can be accomplished by utilizing low-cost manipulatives. While this may seem to be a small component of functional ability, it should not be overlooked. Research indicates that loss of agility in the feet and toes contributes significantly to diminished balance (Perkins-Carpenter, 1991; Spirduso, 1995).

Special attention also should be placed on helping frail seniors overcome the fear of injury. Many frail seniors perceive exercise as potentially harmful, and may in fact have been injured in the past trying to perform inappropriate exercise. Pre-assessments and attention to their personal needs and objectives will help you define program content and objectives that are easily attainable. Success in movement is essential to help frail seniors gain confidence in their ability to be physically active without injury. Refer to Table 6.3 for programming appropriate for frail seniors.

Physically Independent

This category of older adults ranges from individuals who are barely functionally independent, maintaining lifestyles that ask very little of them physically, to seniors who are fairly active, but are not engaged in exercise, work or recreation that keeps them physically "fit." Physically independent seniors need exercise that helps them maintain and improve their physical function, remain independent and prevent illness, disability or injury that could lead to physical frailty. Exercise programming for independent seniors should focus on muscular strength, endurance and flexibility, joint range of motion, balance, coordination and cardiovascular endurance.

Identifying Needs

For an exercise to be considered aerobic it must have the capacity to improve cardiovascular conditioning. Therefore, a chair aerobics class for independent seniors must include an aerobic component. For many clients this can be accomplished through vigorous movement of the arms and the legs. Exercises such as rhythmic knee lifts and kicks to the front and sides, as well as frequently standing up from and sitting down on a chair can be a part of that aerobic component. Chair "dancing" using continuous rhythmic movement of the arms and legs in set patterns also can be a fun way to achieve aerobic conditioning.

Another primary goal is to educate the physically independent senior on the importance of prevention of functional loss, thus motivating them to significantly increase their health and fitness reserves (Barry & Eathorne, 1994; Carter et al., 1991; Resnick, 1991; Schilke, 1991; Shephard, 1993).

One way to do this is to make your program's wellness and fitness messages personally relevant to your clients. For example, if the messages your program gives are all exercise-based, those individuals who have always thought of themselves as non-exercisers will likely find the messages irrelevant. A large number of older adults (especially older women) do not consider themselves the exercise/fitness type. Therefore, the exercise and wellness messages you relay should focus on topics such as maintaining bone strength to combat the effects of osteoporosis, and maintaining leg strength to prevent falls and retain the ability to walk, climb stairs, golf and enjoy travel. In short, messages related to maintaining an independent lifestyle are most appropriate. These messages are relevant to the older adult whether they consider themselves an exerciser or non-exerciser. Refer to

Table 6.4

Programming for the Physically Independent

✓ chair aerobics

✓ low-impact aerobics

✓ modified line dancing and folk dancing

✓ water aerobics

✓ lap swimming

✓ walking programs

✓ circuit training

✓ strength training

✓ recreational activities

✓ Tai Chi

✓ stretching

✓ relaxation

Table 6.5

Programming for the Physically Fit

✓ low-impact aerobics

✓ line dancing and folk dancing

✓ water aerobics

✓ lap swimming

✓ walking programs

✓ circuit training

✓ resistance training

✓ recreational activities

✓ Tai Chi

✓ yoga

✓ stretching

✓ relaxation

✓ sports and games (softball, volleyball, etc.)

Table 6.4 for activities appropriate for physically independent seniors.

Physically Fit

Physically fit older adults require exercise programming that maintains their level of fitness, which in turn allows them to live an active independent lifestyle, work in their chosen professions, and/or participate in a wide range of recreational activities. Programming should focus on muscular strength, endurance and flexibility, joint range of motion, balance, coordination, agility, and cardiovascular endurance. The primary goal in working with Physically fit seniors is to provide them with current, health information and various opportunities to maintain their level of fitness.

Identifying Needs

This group of seniors is generally very self-motivated. They have already determined that physical activity is important to their quality of life. Therefore, your focus will be on

providing convenient and safe "maintenance" programming that address each component of fitness. Emphasize safety because many physically fit seniors are motivated to keep doing more and more without regard for safety. Education on the benefits of appropriate exercise intensity, as well as the risks of inappropriate intensity, is important. Again, it is necessary to emphasize the importance of strength in maintaining functional independence and overall physical fitness. Even those who are involved in water aerobics and low-impact aerobics will notice significant gains in strength through resistance training.

Finally, this group of seniors should be provided with information about the Senior Olympics and other opportunities to challenge their physical abilities. Refer to Table 6.5 for activities appropriate for physically fit seniors.

Physically Elite

Physically elite seniors require exercise programming that helps them maintain their fitness levels, and provides

Table 6.6

Programming for the Physically Elite

✓ low-impact aerobics

✓ line dancing and folk dancing

✓ water aerobics

✓ lap swimming

✓ walking programs (possibly race walking)

✓ circuit training

✓ interval training

✓ resistance training

✓ recreational activities

✓ Tai Chi

✓ yoga

✓ stretching

✓ relaxation

✓ sports and games

✓ sport- or activity-specific training for competition

conditioning for improved performance in competition or in strenuous vocational or recreational activities. Programming should include general conditioning for muscular strength, endurance and flexibility, agility and cardiovascular endurance. It also may include sport- or activity-specific training.

Identifying Needs

Exercise programming for the physically elite often is focused on improving performance in a desired area or areas. Many times this includes intensive strength training. Your role with the physically elite senior is to provide access to appropriate resources and equipment. You also should continue to provide reinforcement of proper exercise intensity and techniques for these highly motivated individuals. Providing the elite senior with information concerning the adverse effects of over-training, and the need for appropriate recovery periods between workouts, will give them the tools to prevent injury while

training and competing. In addition, it is important to provide strategies for addressing injuries if they do occur. Refer to Table 6.6 for a list of activities appropriate for physically elite seniors.

Leveled Programming

Leveled programming refers to offering a range of classes to meet the needs of various levels of functional ability. If you are teaching in a fitness facility, you may only be providing programming for older adults from the upper level of the physically independent category through the physically elite. However, an exercise program at a senior residence facility would require that you provide entry-level activity classes that allow someone in the dependent or frail category to be successful in your program, as well as classes that challenge independent to physically fit older adults. The needs of the physically elite older adult for general conditioning can be met in the upper-level aerobics, circuit and resistance classes. However, the sport- or activity-specific training would be done on an individual basis.

The following pages identify suggestions for appropriate classes using the leveling concept. For detailed descriptions and photographs of specific land- and water-based exercises, please refer to Chapter 5 of this text, and to *Exercise Programming for Older Adults* (Human Kinetics, 1995).

Land-based Programming

Land-based programming includes movement opportunities such as chair exercise, walking, dancing, low-impact aerobics, circuit training, strength training, Tai Chi, yoga, functionally specific stations, recreational activities and a variety of sports and games.

Developing an Individualized Exercise Program

Eleanor is 76 years old with poor vision. She used to enjoy walking several times a week, but hasn't been able to walk alone for almost a year due to fear of falling, and has become sedentary.

Pre-assessments indicate that she has a history of lower-back pain, has lost most of her sight to glaucoma, and is on high blood pressure medication. Physical assessments indicate that her functional status is in the physically frail category. In particular, she is having difficulty getting up from a seated position. In addition, her gait demonstrates a very short stride, flat-footed placement with almost no heel strike, and unsteady balance. The assessments show that this is partly due to weakness in the ankles and legs, and low range of motion in the hips. However, Eleanor's gait abnormality is exaggerated by her extreme fear of falling. She is anxious to regain function, but is fearful of being injured. Eleanor's goals are to rise from a seated position more easily, improve balance and regain the ability to take a walk.

Program Design

Eleanor's most immediate needs are for increased lower-body strength to facilitate a more normal gait pattern and ease in rising from a seated position. This can be accomplished through resistance training on machines and/or with ankle weights. Focus on ankle dorsiflexion (to facilitate an appropriate heel-strike pattern) and quadriceps strength (for rising from a chair). Because of her poor vision, Eleanor will need close supervision in the weight room to facilitate success in movement, alleviate fear and prevent injury.

In addition to strength work, she needs to improve flexibility of the gastrocnemius muscle and the hip extensors to improve her gait pattern.

A secondary need is to address her fear of injury by ensuring that she feels safe in all aspects of the walking movement. Water walking can facilitate balance, coordination and range of motion work, and remove the fear of falling. Land-based balance work also is important for Eleanor to regain the ability to walk for enjoyment, but should be addressed gradually after she has gained confidence and strength. Aerobic conditioning is a secondary concern that should be addressed after she has gained strength and confidence in her ability to exercise without injury. Any aerobic conditioning should be done in water or in a chair, as her poor vision places her at high risk for falling.

Entry Level

Options for entry-level land-based programming include functional-fitness-based chair exercise, resistance training, and the use of home-based (self-directed) exercise brochures. Function-based chair exercise programs consist of exercises that meet the needs of dependent and frail seniors. These exercises help them maintain and improve their ability to perform BADL. Many times, activities programs in senior residence facilities offer a series of games and activities for fun and socialization with little regard for functional needs. Functional-fitness-based programming is equally as important as social activities. Take steps to ensure that your program addresses functional needs and look for ways to add functional tasks to social games and activities whenever possible.

Strength training is such an important part of improving and maintaining function that even very frail older adults can gain significant benefits (Fiatarone, et al., 1994). Resistance training can involve light weights and resistance bands or weight-training machines. After frail seniors become accustomed to the idea of resistance training with light, hand-held weights and resistance bands, allow them to utilize senior-appropriate strength-training machines if possible. Sometimes, when these individuals get a better sense of movement and how it can benefit them, they will be more motivated to utilize strength machines. It is critical for strength-training machines used in senior programming to be "senior appropriate." This means they must be fully adjustable to body size, allow for beginning at minimal weight and for small increments of increased resistance. Keiser air-resistance machines are especially suited to seniors because they meet all these criteria, are non-intimidating and easy to operate.

In skilled nursing facilities, assisted-living facilities and senior housing centers, the home-based exercise concept can be useful. This refers to exercises that focus on maintenance of BADL and can be performed by the individual on a regular basis without supervision. Utilize a variety of simple exercise brochures, each designed to meet the needs of different levels of function. The Permission to M.O.V.E. campaign is particularly useful. It outlines specific strategies for motivating seniors to take an active role in maintaining their functional independence by performing simple, safe exercises daily. This type of programming allows everyone to become involved regardless of whether or not they are motivated to come to a regularly scheduled class. Once you give even very unmotivated older adults the opportunity to move on a regular basis and offer reinforcement for their efforts, they typically become more inclined to further increase their level of physical activity. Some even progress to choosing to participate in structured classes.

Level II

Options for Level II programming include walking, functional-fitness-based station work, more vigorous chair exercise (involving some aerobic conditioning), circuit training, flexibility training and strength training. Walking programs can include walking trails (indoor or outdoor), as well as station formats. Emphasis should not only be placed on getting residents walking, but also on the importance of maintaining or normalizing posture and gait patterns while walking. The stations format allows residents to walk from one functional-fitness station to the next and is advantageous because it is available on a continuous basis. When using the stations format at senior residence facilities, exercises must be chosen carefully to incorporate a level of basic functional ability, posing minimal risks to potentially unsupervised participants.

Chair exercise can incorporate functional fitness activities with a higher level of coordination, flexibility, balance and strength work. In addition, an aerobic phase is gradually added to improve cardiovascular health.

A supervised circuit- or strength-training program also is appropriate at this level. Circuit training involves alternating between a strength machine and an aerobic machine throughout a pre-set circuit. The strength-training program utilizes strength equipment alone with specific goals for improving strength in both the lower and upper body.

Tai Chi also is a good choice for Level II programming. Its slow, controlled movement with concentration on breathing and internalizing balance and coordination is appropriate for older adults. The challenge with Tai Chi may be the pre-conceived idea of what the practice of Tai Chi means. Many older adults relate it to some type of religion and, therefore, are reluctant to become involved with this type of activity. Try incorporating some of the Tai Chi movement techniques into a class they are already comfortable with such as low-impact aerobics. The movements become balance and coordination work rather than formalized Tai Chi training.

Level III

The third level of land-based programming should include activities such as low-impact aerobics, walking or jogging, circuit training, strength training, line and folk dancing, and a variety of recreational activities.

Low-impact aerobic programs should consist of gentle movement to music as a warm-up, continuous, simple movement to music for an aerobics phase, a resistance phase, and a cool-down and stretch phase. One sound approach to a balanced program, for example, includes approximately 10 to 20 minutes of warm-up, coordination and balance work; 20 to 25 minutes of aerobics; and 15 to 20 minutes of cool-down, strengthening and stretching. Focus on safety by weighing the benefits against the risks for each choice. Movement choices and class format also must be structured in a way that allows all clients to feel successful. Your program structure should exhibit simple patterns without complicated combinations, surprise direction changes, or fast cross-over steps that can put clients at risk for a fall. Embrace a teaching style that relays information about what is coming next (i.e., hand signals and voice cueing before a change). In addition, return to simple steps (such as marching in place) often to ensure that all participants are successful in movement at least some of the time, and most are successful the majority of the time. For specific exercise descriptions, please refer to Chapter 5 of this text and *Exercise Programming for Older Adults* in the suggested reading list.

Note that classes such as Tai Chi, circuit training, strength training and functionally specific fitness stations can be used at several levels of programming. With proper supervision, these classes can be structured to simultaneously meet the needs of seniors from a variety of functional ability levels.

Water-based Programming

Water-based programming refers to any activities that are conducted in the water, such as water walking, one-on-one water exercise, water aerobics, water circuit training, games such as water polo, and swimming. Water-based programming at each level can simultaneously meet the needs of seniors at a variety of levels of functional ability. An individual can work as hard or as gently as they choose to in the water. This allows a water aerobics class, for example, to be a gentle workout for some, or a vigorous workout for the person who chooses to resist the water with the arms and lift the knees more quickly and/or higher than average. For detailed descriptions and examples, refer to chapter 5, and *Exercise Programming for Older Adults,* and *Aquatics: The Complete Reference Guide for Aquatic Fitness Professionals* in the suggested reading list.

Entry Level

Entry-level classes in water-based programming include one-on-one water exercise and group or individual water walking. In one-on-one water exercise, an instructor helps a student move through a set of goal-specific exercises in the pool. Water walking engages participants in walking forward, backward and sideways across the pool. Variations are numerous and include using long strides, short strides, cross-over steps, a heel-strike pattern, walking on tip toes, and walking with bent or straight knees. Emphasis can be placed on using these variations to improve coordination and balance. This class also should include a strength segment, a flexibility segment and a cool-down and relaxation segment. Water walking classes usually are designed to improve strength, range of motion, coordination and balance for older adults who are not ready for an aerobic program, or who simply prefer a gentle workout.

Level II

The second level of water-based programming includes a Water Aerobics Level I class. This class commonly includes a 20- to 25-minute warm-up; a range-of-motion, coordination and strength phase; a 15- to 20-minute cardiovascular conditioning (aerobic) phase; and a 20- to 25-minute cool-down and stretch phase. Another option within this level of programming is to provide an opportunity for those who enjoy lap swimming.

Level III

The third level includes Water Aerobics Level II, which generally uses the same format as Level I, except the aerobic segment is increased to 20 to 25 minutes. It also could include more repetitions or more difficult exercises in the strength segment, and more complicated coordination work. It is still important, however, to provide a balanced class with 15 to 20 minutes of warm-up; range-of-motion, strength and coordination work; and 15 to 20 minutes of cool-down and stretching. Lap swimming also is appropriate for this level of programming.

Warm-up

Regardless of the mode of exercise chosen (i.e., land, water, chair), never begin a senior exercise class with aggressive stretching. Seniors tend to have diminished flexibility of the tendons, ligaments and muscles, resulting in a higher potential for muscle and tendon strain and tears (Spirduso, 1995). Begin

your classes with a combination of gentle continuous movement and easy range-of-motion activities to increase circulation. Gentle static stretching and preparatory stretching also can be part of a senior warm-up. When incorporating static stretching into a warm-up, have seniors stretch to a comfortable range of motion and hold that stretch. Stretching to the point of mild discomfort for the purpose of increasing flexibility should only be performed at the end of a class when muscles are thoroughly warmed.

The warm-up phase is a good place to teach any new movement sequence you plan to use later in the aerobic phase of class. This gives students a chance to try the movement slowly and gain confidence before attempting to execute the movement in time with the music during aerobics. Have your students perform the ranges of motion they will be performing during the aerobics phase. For example, if you plan to push the arms overhead during the aerobic phase then it is a good idea to perform the same action more slowly during the warm-up.

Safe Movements

When choosing movement possibilities, weigh the risks against the benefits of each type of exercise. Choose smooth rather than jerky arm movements, and completed movements rather than choppy or jerky starts and stops. Smooth, complete movements reduce the risk of joint stress and injury to participants. In land-based exercise classes, low-impact movements are the only appropriate choice for an older adult class, since high-impact movements pose an unacceptably high level of risk. Simple movements and movement combinations are safer and promote self-confidence by allowing the participants to be successful in movement. Many seniors have lost a significant amount of coordination if they have not been participating regularly in a coordination- promoting activity. Therefore, rapid changes of direction and complicated movement patterns increase both anxiety and the danger of falling. They also decrease self-esteem and the overall enjoyment of those who are unsuccessful in the movement. While keeping movements simple, you must also make an effort to use a variety of movement combinations, music and teaching formations to keep classes fun and interesting. In strength-training classes be very conscientious about ensuring proper body alignment and exercise techniques. Teach clients to perform resistance work through their pain-free range of motion. In addition, be aware of machines that allow hyperextension or hyperflexion of the joints, and make sure seniors know how to adjust these machines to prevent joint stress and injury.

Managing Aerobic Training Risks

Due to the high incidence of cardiovascular dysfunction in the older adult population, it is important to use a variety of methods to help ensure that your participants are exercising at an appropriate aerobic level. This can be achieved by determining individual target heart-rate zones, using the rating of perceived exertion scale and frequent heart-rate checks. A combination of methods will help your students learn how intense their exercise should be.

Determining Intensity

As an instructor, it is your job to make sure each individual participating in cardiovascular conditioning activities knows their individually determined target heart-rate range. Research shows that even moderate- to low-intensity aerobic exercise provides a training benefit for many seniors (Barry & Eathorne, 1994). Use the Karvonen formula for

your students without heart disease and vary the intensity of your aerobics from the low end (50 percent) to the high end (75 percent) of the aerobic range throughout the workout. To facilitate this varied intensity, carefully arrange to play your aerobic music at alternating tempos within 120 to 140 beats per minute. For example, after the warm-up phase, arrange music to play slow (120 bpm), medium (130 bpm), fast (140 bpm), medium (130 bpm), slow (120 bpm), medium (130 bpm), fast (140 bpm) and then medium (130 bpm). This method provides aerobic training benefits while reducing the risks associated with bringing seniors to the higher end of their aerobic range and having them stay there the entire aerobic phase.

Make certain that each senior knows their target heart-rate range and what their 10-second count should be. To effectively use the target heart-rate range, use a simple and consistent method to check heart rates. This helps ensure that all class members can successfully find and count their pulse. It is a good practice to use the same cues each time you take an exercise pulse rate. Make the cues clear and direct: *Stop and find your pulse.* Then pause for two to three seconds, and say, *Ready, start,* having them count for 10 seconds, and then say, *Stop.* As soon as the 10-second count is completed, participants can march in place while each person tells you their heart rate. If you practice taking exercise and recovery pulse rates with your students, it will only take moments for each heart-rate check. When they all feel comfortable and confident with the procedure, they will provide you with more accurate feedback on their heart rates.

Your senior students with known heart disease should exercise at a heart rate recommended by their physician that corresponds to a comfortable exertion. It is critical to note that medications that regulate the heart rate invalidate target heart-rate calculations.

Therefore, you must know which of your students take medication. Clients on this type of medication should rely on perceived exertion ratings. Exercisers should learn to work at a level they can identify as somewhere between moderate to moderately hard during the aerobic phase of the class. While exercising, an individual should be able to carry on a conversation without gasping for air. Even clients who are not on medications that alter heart rates should learn to use the rating of perceived exertion method since it provides one more safeguard to maintaining an appropriate exercise intensity, and provides important information about how an individual is responding to exercise that day. The body's response to exercise is affected by many things, including heat, cold, medications, stress or illness. Due to many outside factors, an individual may be exercising below their target zone, but feel as though they are working moderately hard to hard. Giving as much importance to the rate of perceived exertion as to the calculated target heart-rate zone helps to ensure that participants are exercising at a safe level that is in line with their body's response to exercise that day.

Monitoring Intensity

Again, it is a good practice to check heart rates after the warm-up since this will tell clients how their body is responding to exercise that day. Monitor exercise intensity frequently by checking heart rates twice during the aerobic phase and asking each person to tell you their 10-second count or their perceived exertion rating. This only takes a matter of seconds during a class, and gives you immediate feedback to determine if someone is exercising at a potentially unsafe rate. It also continually reinforces the concept that appropriate exercise intensity is essential to safe, effective exercise.

In low-impact aerobics, the circle formation used for variety and interest also provides a valuable opportunity for you to examine each individual's response to the exercise intensity. Look for signs of overexertion such as a flushed face and unusually rapid breathing. You also can ask everyone how they are doing, how the temperature in the room feels, and casually give someone the talk test by asking them a direct question requiring more than a one-word answer.

At the end of the aerobic phase, check their final exercise heart rate. Have clients reduce exercise intensity (walking slowly or a similar activity) for one minute, then take their recovery pulse for 10 seconds. Ask each student how many beats they decreased in the one-minute recovery period. If you have a student whose pulse does not decrease after one minute, take their pulse again one minute later to determine if it has decreased. Failure of the heart to noticeably recover after aerobic exercise can be an indication of a variety of problems. This individual should be monitored throughout the rest of the class to determine if their heart rate is responding. Clients whose heart rate does not return to their pre-exercise level five to 10 minutes after completing the exercise should be referred to their physician.

During the cool-down phase, ask each student, regardless of whether or not they are on heart-rate medication, to indicate their perceived exertion rating. This will help your students begin to understand how they feel when they are exercising within their target heart-rate zone.

Recording Exercise Intensity

Write each student's predetermined 10-second count, or an indication of reliance on the perceived exertion rating, next to their names on the role sheet or a chart for easy referral. An effective strategy is to keep a record of each student's exercise heart rate, recovery heart rate and perceived exertion rating for every exercise period during the first several weeks of class. Refer to Figure 6.2 for a sample chart that can be used in this manner. Recording these figures will help you to become familiar with each individual's response to exercise and alert you to potential problems such as excessively high exercise heart rates or failure of the heart to recover after one minute. It also will help reinforce to your students the importance of monitoring their exercise intensity with both the target heart rate and rating of perceived exertion. After you become familiar with your class members and their responses to exercise, continue to ask each participant for these numbers even if you no longer take the time to record them.

Attention to Detail

When developing programs for older adults, a little attention to detail goes a long way toward effectively meeting their needs. Refer to Chapter 5 for movement strategies to meet the needs and objectives of your particular class population. However, regardless of the strategies or the level of programming used, you must understand the importance of fostering a social atmosphere in your classes. This begins with your ability to project a friendly, interested attitude to each class member. Learning participants' names, greeting them as they enter class, introducing new participants to others in the group, and checking on regulars who miss class are all effective ways to show concern for individuals in the group. Enjoying the social interaction is consistently listed as one of the top reasons seniors continue to attend group exercise classes, so look for ways to encourage and support social interaction among participants. Vary the class formation from facing front to lines facing each other, to arranging the class in a circle, to provide opportunities for participants to exchange comments and smiles while they exercise. During a low-impact aerobics class, for example, the circle formation often results in someone sharing a joke or something that happened on the way to class.

Another aspect of making a class "senior friendly" is to give special attention to the tempo and type of music. Somewhere in the range of 120 to 140 beats per minute works well for the aerobic portion of the class. Music should have a steady, easily distinguishable beat, with simple instrumentals and mid-range vocals. Slower music (that also has a steady beat) works well for the warm-up. Music for the cool-down

FIGURE 6.2

	Date																
Name		EHR/R	RPE	EHR/R	RPE	EHR/R	RPE	EHR/R	RPE	EHR/R	RPE	EHR/R	RPE	EHR/R	RPE	EHR/R	RPE

EHR=exercise heart rate; R=recovery heart rate; RPE=rating of perceived exertion
Van Norman, Kay, (1995), Exercise Programming for Older Adults, Human Kinetics.

and stretch phase of the class can be similar to the warm-up music or it can be of the easy-listening or relaxation variety. The type of music used is just as important as the tempo. Music that was popular during the time your class participants were young adults may bring back good memories and increase their enjoyment. Ask your seniors what music they like. Many will be happy to suggest favorite records and tapes to you. Inappropriate music can result in a very unenthusiastic group or no group at all! There are currently a number of music companies that are producing senior exercise recordings. You also can pick up some great "oldies" selections from most music stores.

Music volume also is an important consideration. Do not assume that since many older adults have diminished hearing, you should turn the volume up loudly. Most seniors dislike loud music, and those with some degree of deafness will not necessarily benefit from the increased volume. Seniors with uncorrected impairments will have a very difficult time hearing any of your instruction because of the loud music. Those with hearing aids may be most troubled by loud music because the aid magnifies all sounds, producing an uncomfortable mixture of music, voices and background noise. The most effective strategy is to play the music at a moderate volume, watch for your students' response, and ask them how well they can hear the rhythm. Soon you will be able to easily recognize the volume appropriate to each class.

Be aware that when you are giving a lot of verbal instruction, such as explaining a new exercise, it is best to turn the music off so that it does not compete with your voice. Trying to hear new instructions over music can be very frustrating for older clients, especially those who are new to the class and already anxious about learning new movements and patterns.

Participant Recruitment

Before developing a plan for recruiting participants it is important to determine who you are trying to recruit. As outlined in the beginning of this chapter, the term "senior exerciser" encompasses individuals from a broad range of functional abilities and exercise needs. Facility, staffing and financial considerations will largely determine the type of programming you can provide and, thus, the type of senior you target.

Facility

Facility type, size and location, as well as accessibility for anyone with functional impairments, are significant factors in determining who you will be programming for. The type of equipment available for classes and the existing atmosphere of a facility also are important considerations.

Type

Facility type is an obvious consideration. Exercise programming for skilled nursing and assisted-living facilities would consist of classes primarily for older adults in the dependent and frail categories. Senior residence facilities catering to the independent older adult and senior citizen centers may require exercise programming that meets the needs of the frail to physically fit senior. Fitness facilities catering to the general public would most likely provide programming for seniors from the independent to the more physically fit and elite categories of function.

Size

Facility size largely determines your programming options. Sizes range from very large facilities with access to extensive equipment, to small fitness centers with very little equipment. In senior housing complexes, an exercise facility can range from one small room to having access to a whole wellness center complete with a swimming pool, weight room and aerobics room.

Location and Accessibility

The facility's location also is important. Facilities in a central area that can easily be reached on foot or by public transportation have the advantage of attracting older adults who no longer drive. In contrast, hard-to-reach facilities, regardless of the amenities offered, will be under-utilized by a large percentage of seniors. Similarly, facilities in high-crime areas are not likely to attract a large percentage of senior participants.

Equally as important as an accessible location is the accessibility of the facility itself to those with mobility impairments. Parking areas that are far from the building or facilities with excessive stairs make it difficult for many seniors in the lower range of the independent category to participate in programs. In areas where snow and ice are a problem, poorly maintained parking lots and sidewalks also serve as a barrier to participation. Parking and environmental obstacles can make it impossible for older adults from the frail and dependent categories to access your program.

Equipment and Facility Systems

Equipment options within the facility are a consideration when programming for seniors. Weight-lifting machines should be fully adjustable to body size and allow for increasing resistance by small increments ($2\frac{1}{2}$ pounds or less). Weight machines without these features not only pose an increased risk of injury to older adults, but can be especially intimidating to many older women as well.

Exercise facilities lacking appropriate heating or cooling systems can pose a hazard to seniors whose bodies often do not regulate heat as efficiently as

those of younger adults. Evaluating these aspects of the facility in advance allows you to make the necessary adjustments for safe programming.

Atmosphere

One often-overlooked aspect of facility appropriateness is the existing atmosphere within a facility. Some facilities are a hang out for the body beautiful set, or muscle men and women. These types of facilities do not provide a comfortable atmosphere for older adults, especially those who are trying exercise for the first time in many years and already feel like they don't belong there.

Another aspect of appropriateness concerns the times the facility is available for programming. To some degree, the times of your program determine the type of seniors you will attract. Some seniors are early risers and love to get up and complete their exercise before proceeding with the rest of their day. Others possess the attitude that *I'm retired, and don't want to get up early any more!* To reach the largest percentage of seniors, offer both early morning and early afternoon classes if possible. The most critical component of scheduling is that it is consistent, allowing seniors to rely on a specific time and day for their program choice.

Evaluating the advantages and limitations of a facility helps you identify what types of programs are appropriate within that environment, and for which segments of the senior population you can provide safe and effective programming.

Staffing

Staff training and staff/participant ratios also must be a primary consideration when determining the level of programming you will provide. Meeting the needs of clients in the physically frail to physically dependent categories requires a highly trained staff with a thorough knowledge of limitations, as well as appropriate expectations for this group. The staff/participant ratio must be small enough to provide close supervision. This type of programming is most common to senior housing, such as assisted-living facilities and skilled nursing facilities.

Programs striving to meet the needs of the independent, physically fit and elite categories of seniors are most common to community-based fitness facilities. Programs for these segments of the population allow for larger staff-to-participant ratios. However, as the instructor, you must be aware of the range of abilities common to seniors within these three categories. Of special importance is the broad range of functional abilities and limitations of seniors classified as functionally independent. Some functionally independent seniors are very close to being physically fit. However, others will walk into your class with no obvious functional impairments but, in fact, have significantly diminished levels of balance, coordination, strength and flexibility. This is the group of older adults that is at the highest risk for injury. Administering appropriate pre-assessments, and using senior-safe activities and teaching styles throughout your programming is an important safeguard for preventing injuries.

Cost

Facility and staffing considerations are largely responsible for determining the cost of senior programming. Many times, the cost of the program plays a vital role in determining who will be attending your classes. Evaluating population demographics in your area with regard to numbers of seniors, average incomes and percentage of seniors within each economic category will help you determine realistic expectations for program recruitment.

Marketing Strategies

After careful consideration of all the elements described above, you can determine which segments of the senior population you can provide programming for. Once these market segments are identified, begin developing marketing strategies.

A large part of marketing your program is developing cooperative relationships with other individuals and organizations that work daily to provide a variety of services to the seniors in your community. Develop mutually beneficial relationships with senior services and health professional networks in your area.

Senior Services

A very beneficial step you can take to market a senior exercise program is to become an integral part of the senior services network in your community. This includes senior centers, area agencies on aging, county offices on aging and a wide range of senior support services that vary dramatically from community to community. It is a good practice to make both general information about the benefits of exercise and specific information about your program easily available throughout this senior services network. Look for ways to include information about this network in your own promotional materials, such as the availability of a senior transportation service as a way to get to your program. A safe and effective exercise program will be a welcome addition to the network of services for seniors.

Health Professionals

An important part of your network should be area physicians, physical therapists and orthopedic specialists. Utilize their expertise and request their input on program components. Seek their advice on such things as the level of aerobic conditioning appropriate to seniors with heart- and lung-related restrictions, and on the safety of specific exercises for special muscle and joint conditions. Establish a relationship of trust and reliability within this network. This is an ongoing process that takes time and careful attention to detail, but offers a great deal in return. Adequately involving area health professionals increases your program's safety and credibility. It also increases participation through direct referrals from these health professionals (Van Norman, 1995). Current literature from numerous health-related disciplines strongly supports the belief that the right kind of exercise can improve many aspects of health (Spirduso, 1995; Barry & Eathorne, 1994; Schilke, 1991; Shephard, 1993; Chandler, 1996). Therefore, if area health professionals know you have a safe, effective program, they will be motivated to refer patients to your classes.

If you live in an area with close access to a college or university, it is a good practice to include its health and fitness professionals in your network. This relationship can be mutually beneficial, offering you access to current information in the field of exercise and aging, and offering research faculty an opportunity to involve your group in appropriate research projects.

Focusing Your Marketing Efforts

When developing a marketing strategy for your program, you must obviously consider where to focus your marketing efforts. If you are programming for a residence facility, your market is already established since it is usually limited to on-site residents. In this instance, you must identify the range of functional abilities and needs within the resident population, and analyze how facility operations, such as meal schedules and medication distribution,

support or restrict implementation of exercise programs. When developing programming that meets functional needs, remember to identify and program for your clients' interests. The compliance rate among seniors engaging in self-chosen activities is significantly higher than for those engaging in non-choice activities (Mills et al., 1997).

In community-based programs, you must find the senior consumer. Analyze where seniors do business, where their health needs are met, and where they congregate socially in your community. After locating the senior consumer, develop a marketing plan to ensure your materials are readily available to them.

Businesses

An effective strategy for marketing is to identify businesses that cater to older adults, such as clothing and shoe stores, gift shops, book stores, novelty shops, and barbers or hair designers. Look for businesses taking special care to be friendly and accommodating to seniors. Determine which restaurants draw a large number of older customers. Some restaurants cater to older adults with discounts and senior nights, offering additional discounts and extra special service. Some older cafés may be longtime favorites of seniors. In addition, identify a grocery store that is within walking distance to senior housing or shopping complexes offering one-stop shopping. Many seniors without personal transportation frequent stores where they can be dropped off for a few hours to take care of all their needs in one place (Van Norman, 1995).

Healthcare Providers

Consider where a high percentage of the older adults in your community are likely to have their health needs met. Seniors consume a high percentage of prescription drugs sold, so it is important to identify which drugstores cater to seniors. Look for one with a convenient location or one offering delivery service. If possible, identify the doctors who have a large senior clientele. They will include internists, family practice doctors, those who specialize in arthritis and doctors who have been in the community for many years. Most doctors' offices have a bulletin board where notices can be posted. If you have a good relationship with area physicians, many will go a step further and place posters in examining rooms or hand out your materials when recommending exercise (Van Norman, 1995).

Social and Recreation Network

Determine where the seniors in your community socialize and recreate. Senior centers, social clubs, city recreation centers, golf courses, bingo parlors, special community events and night clubs with social dance music are likely choices. Determining where seniors go to enjoy themselves will help you target your marketing. A large number of seniors also socialize through volunteer work. Identify community organizations specifically designed to offer volunteer work, as well as other volunteer opportunities such as museums, hospitals and churches.

Developing Relevant Messages

As previously discussed in this chapter, messages designed to reach potential senior clients must be relevant to them personally. Messages about your program that focus primarily on exercise and broad terms of wellness will only speak to that small percentage of seniors who consider themselves "exercisers." Therefore, when developing your media messages, determine who you are trying to reach and what issues pertaining to physical function and health are relevant to them. Since the largest number of seniors can be classified as functionally independent, it

seems appropriate that many of your messages should focus on maintaining an independent lifestyle.

Highlighting Activities of Interest

An additional aspect of recruiting senior exercise participants is determining which types of activities they are most likely to participate in (Mills et al., 1996). A large number of senior programs consist of one or a variety of group-based classes led by an instructor. These programs attract seniors who either prefer group exercise or don't really have a preference for exercising (group or individual). The benefit of social interaction in group settings has been consistently reported (Spirduso, 1995). A recent study, however, points out that there also is a significant percentage of seniors who prefer to exercise on an individual basis (Mills et al., 1997). This study reflects that a similar degree of individual preferences for type of exercise appears in all age categories. Regardless of age, some people prefer group activities while others prefer individualized ones. This is a very simple but important point to consider when developing your programs and beginning recruitment procedures.

To reach those who prefer individualized experiences, your recruitment materials must highlight ways in which this type of activity will be used in your program. Note that activities suggested for meeting the needs of different levels of functional ability include both individualized and group activities. Some seniors may participate in group activities but will appreciate the opportunity to work individually; others may simply not participate because of a lack of individualized programming. An effective strategy for reaching these seniors is to ensure that your promotional messages emphasize how activities such as circuit training, strength training and station formats can be either group-oriented or individualized. Even walking programs can be individualized. They can promote walking together at a set time and place, but also can be structured to allow individuals to walk on their own, keeping track of their progress through a cumulative minutes or miles program. Their progress can be recorded both individually and in the group's record.

Using the Media

Newspapers, television and radio can play a role in helping you reach the senior consumer. Newspaper editors have found that their most loyal readers are the older adult population and are responding with a significant increase in the coverage of aging issues that are personally relevant to seniors. Older television viewers' preference for news, sports, talk shows and classic movies has begun to change the programming focus of cable television from entertainment only to a mix of entertainment, news and lifestyle. The radio industry also is taking notice that older listeners are significantly more likely to listen to all-news formats, news/talk formats, easy-listening and nostalgia programs.

These are important considerations when determining where to spend advertising dollars and how to utilize the media's focus on senior issues to promote your program. Television footage of seniors exercising in your program and personal interviews with seniors who want to talk about what exercise has done for them personally, work very well to generate interest in your program.

Compliance and Motivation

Many seniors are motivated to begin an exercise program due to a physician's advice. Many others will be motivated by a noticeable loss of physical abilities and a desire to regain full function (Strain, 1996). Regardless of their

reasoning, they will join a program that addresses their individual needs, and be motivated to continue a program if they experience noticeable improvements in physical capacities or an overall feeling of well-being (Barry & Eathorne, 1994). If you have a well-balanced program, clients will achieve noticeable results. Solicit feedback from your group on how they feel about their progress. Determine what improvements they notice in endurance, strength, flexibility, overall mobility and well-being. Refer to Chapter 4 for using appropriate pre- and post-assessments to track an individual's progress.

Goals and Rewards

An effective strategy for motivating seniors is to develop a program of mini-goals and a system of rewards, prizes and mini-celebrations for reaching those goals. Chapter 2 includes a discussion of specific strategies for setting goals. Consider giving T-shirts and certificates of honor for regular attendance. Efforts to reward participation can provide that extra motivation a person sometimes needs to make exercise part of their healthy lifestyle.

When developing rewards systems it is important to make goals achievable for all participants, regardless of functional ability. A goal of walking 10 miles per week, for example, may be easy for some seniors, but impossible for others. Therefore, keeping track of the time spent walking may be more appropriate if you are providing programming for seniors from a range of functional abilities. Using the time-spent format works well for many forms of physical activity, including seated functional-based work and vigorous aerobics. Similarly, having a time limit to reach rewards (one month, for example) may pose difficulty for some seniors. Design your goal system so that rewards are given for reaching benchmarks of time spent, regardless of how long it takes an individual to reach the benchmark. You can combine this basic reward system with a series of extra rewards for additional accomplishments.

Finally, when designing your goals and rewards, you need to give some thought to how much time it will take to track or record individual progress. If the recording of individual progress is left to the instructor, it becomes a time-intensive project. Consider developing a system that allows each individual to record their own progress in an individual exercise log, a group chart, or both.

Social and Emotional Motivation

A healthy lifestyle involves physical, mental and social/emotional well-being. It is beneficial to design a program that strives to improve as many of these areas as possible. Setting a positive tone within your program begins with the first phone call a senior consumer makes to your program. Project professionalism in a friendly, interested manner, providing the information that is requested, and asking important questions about the caller in return. Ask them about their current level of physical condition, if they are now, or have recently been involved, in a regular exercise program, and what health and fitness goals they hope to achieve. It also is important to ask them what types of activities they are most interested in, and which they feel most comfortable participating in.

There are many reasons why someone may attend an exercise program. They may wish to improve their aerobic condition, strength in their legs and/or upper body, balance and coordination to prevent falls, or flexibility for decreased pain and increased mobility. Their goals may also be less specific, such as improving their overall appearance and health, or improving their social life. Knowing what a person is hoping to

accomplish will help you determine how your program can best meet their needs. This exchange of information should be conversational rather than interrogative. When you have gathered the necessary information, explain how your program can help them accomplish their goals. If you offer a variety of classes, suggest the ones that will best meet their needs. Be prepared to visit with the client as long as necessary to obtain the needed information and to get to know a little something about the person who is about to become part of your family of senior exercisers.

Making this first phone call to inquire about an exercise program is a big step for many older adults. A large part of your marketing program is designed to initiate this first step. If a potential client's phone call is met with impatience or indifference, they will not be motivated to visit or participate in your program.

When the senior arrives in class for the first time, give them a warm welcome and introduction to the class to generate a feeling of belonging among participants. Knowing clients' names and something specific about each one, such as a special interest or talent, reinforces a sense of belonging. Whenever possible, take time to visit before and after classes with your students. Also make time within the class for exchanges between instructor and participants and among participants. Generating a feeling of belonging to something special is key to motivating seniors to continue an exercise program (Van Norman, 1995).

Equipment: Balancing Needs with Cost

Senior exercise programs housed within an existing fitness facility, university setting or large wellness center within a senior housing complex will usually allow access to a wide range of equipment. It is ideal to have weight machines, aerobic machines, pool access and specialized fitness rooms to support program development and implementation. However, a large percentage of senior exercise programs exist within a small fitness facility, a designated corner of a senior citizens' center or a senior housing facility's activities room. Either in the absence of equipment or just for fun and variety, there are a number of inexpensive items that can be utilized in an exercise class for older adults.

Tactile Manipulatives

Koosh™ balls and gel balls are wonderful props to use in chair exercise classes. They are light and easy to handle, have an interesting feel and can be easily squeezed in one hand. Another advantage is that they are easy to toss up in the air and catch, as they will not bounce off a person's hands like a tennis or foam ball. Koosh balls and gel balls rolled up and down the legs and arms, and in between the hands, provide tactile stimulation and help increase circulation, which can be especially beneficial in classes for dependent or frail seniors. These balls can also be used to exercise the feet, and can be rolled back and forth with the sole of the foot to provide a wonderful foot massage. The participants can attempt to pick up the Koosh ball from the floor by gripping it with their toes, promoting foot and toe mobility. You can also have seniors pinch the gel balls between their fingers and thumb to improve pinch grip. Lack of foot mobility is identified as a contributor to falls, and pinch grip is closely associated with the ability to perform BADL (Spirduso, 1995).

Even something as simple as a newspaper can be used to improve hand agility. Have seniors hold up a half-sheet of newspaper by the corner with their right hand, and use the fingers of that hand to draw the newspaper into a ball. Then have seniors transfer the newspaper ball into their left hand and use only that hand to smooth out the newspaper ball.

Sponges of various sizes and shapes also can be used to squeeze and grip. Place a large sponge under the armpit, squeezing it flat against the body to work the shoulder and upper-arm muscles; or squeeze it between the knees to work the inner thigh muscles. Sponges can also be used as a prop to contract the abdominal muscles by asking seniors to flatten the sponge between their back and the chair back. Clients also may squeeze or wring the sponges in their hands, or roll and squeeze them with their feet and toes. They also are a good prop for promoting ankle flexion. Have seniors place their toes on the sponge (heels on the floor), and then raise the ball of the foot and toes off of the sponge by flexing the ankle. Utilizing the sponge as a prop gives seniors a concrete image of what it means to flex the ankle, and often results in increased performance of the desired action.

Manipulatives that Promote Range of Motion

An object such as a wooden dowel, old necktie or other piece of cloth can be used as an aid in promoting range of motion. For example, have seniors grasp a wooden dowel, tie or cloth in both hands and press it out in front of them (at shoulder level, horizontal to the floor), then straight overhead, and gently behind the head. Using this type of manipulative helps many seniors perform a larger range of motion than is achieved with simple verbal instructions of *raise your arms overhead* or *pull your shoulder blades together*.

By focusing on the specific functional needs of older adults, you can identify everyday items that can be used to promote these functions.

Resistance Exercise Equipment

In the absence of weight machines, resistance bands and hand-held weights are useful for promoting strength. In addition, they are valuable for providing entry-level resistance work for those unable or unwilling to use the machines.

Resistance bands are stretchy bands that come in a variety of strengths, from light to heavy resistance. They can be ordered from most fitness supply catalogs, and are used to help develop both upper- and lower-body strength. A resistance band approximately 3 feet long works well for both upper- and lower-body exercises. When working on upper-body strength, use care to keep the elbow next to, or in front of, the body. Having the elbow behind the body while performing strength moves involving the shoulder joint can create impingement of the shoulder joint, a painful condition for a senior exerciser. In addition, ensure that your participants understand that the wrist must be held in a neutral position (not hyperflexed or hyperextended) when performing the exercises. Refer to Chapter 3 for additional high-risk exercises and Chapter 5 for specific exercise sequences.

Light ankle/wrist weights also are very useful for chair-based senior exercise classes. Ankle/wrist weights are more versatile than hand-held weights because they can be strapped on the ankle or around the wrist, or held in the hand. Variable weights can be used individually or added together for increased resistance, and work well for most seniors involved in chair exercise. Strength-training studies have demonstrated that even very frail seniors can safely participate in resistance training (Fiatarone, 1994). These studies utilized strength-training machines and had participants perform sets lifting 80 percent of the maximum they could lift one time. While you may not have access to weight-training machines, resistance bands and weights provide opportunities for participants to challenge and improve their strength. In the absence of any financial resources for resistance equipment, you can use milk jugs or plastic soda bottles filled with sand, or other household items such as soup cans, for resistance. When using these types of items, strongly emphasize the importance of proper joint alignment, as holding onto these objects may be awkward.

Water-based Equipment

There is a variety of water-based equipment used to aid in flotation, including water bells, long foam noodles and kick boards. Water bells and foam noodles are easy to hold in the hand and can be placed under the armpits. This is advantageous in programs serving seniors with severe arthritis in the hands. In the absence of a budget for equipment, milk jugs also work well for flotation. It is not advisable for seniors with severe arthritis to use the jugs, however, as gripping the small handles can aggravate their condition.

There also is a growing variety of resistance equipment designed for strength work in water. Water gloves and hand-held paddles can be used for upper-body exercises. Using ankle weights in the water for older adult classes is not recommended because it is difficult to monitor proper alignment under water. Adding weight while performing exercises increases the risk of injury to participants who are not always performing the exercises with proper alignment. This is a case where it is useful to weigh the benefits of adding the weights against the possible risks.

Conclusion

Exercise programming for older adults is a rapidly growing field within the exercise and wellness professions. The knowledge base of research and practice is growing daily. In addition to available resources, there also are growing networks of professionals focused on senior exercise. Providing programming for this population is both challenging and rewarding. The challenge lies in carefully planning programs that balance the special needs of seniors with their fitness needs, and in keeping pace with the ongoing research relevant to this field. As an exercise instructor for older adults, you have a responsibility to continue reviewing research in the area of exercise and aging, and to determine what it means to you the practitioner. In addition, it is beneficial to participate in the growing networks of senior exercise specialists to share program ideas and strengthen your professionalism.

Those who work with older adults, from the physically dependent through physically elite categories, can also gain a true sense of satisfaction. It is very rewarding working with dependent and frail seniors to help them maintain the dignity that comes with self-care, and to help guide independent older adults to a lifestyle that includes the physical activity necessary to maintain a positive quality of life. Working with the physically fit and elite older adults to help them attain a goal can also provide a sense of accomplishment, as well as wonderful role models for the aging. Few fields provide such an opportunity for positively impacting the lives of others and, at the same time, gaining personal inspiration.

References

Barry, H.C. & Eathorne, S.W. (1994). Exercise and aging: Issues for the practitioner. *Sports Medicine,* 78, 2, 357-376.

Binder, E.F., Brown, M., Craft, S., Schechtman, K.B. & Birge, S.J. (1994). Effects of a group exercise program on risk factors for falls in frail older adults. *Journal of Aging and Physical Activity,* 2, 25-37.

Carter, W.B., Elward, K., Malmgren, J., Martin, M.L. & Larson, E. (1991). Participation of older adults in health programs and research: A critical review of the literature. *The Gerontologist,* 31, 5, 584-592.

Chandler, J.M. (1996). Understanding the relationship between strength and mobility in frail older persons: A review of the literature. *Topics in Geriatric Rehabilitation,* 11, 3, 20-37.

Chandler, J.M., Duncan, P.W., Sanders, L. & Studenski, S. (1996). The fear of falling syndrome: Relationship to falls, physical performance and activities of daily living in frail older persons. *Topics in Geriatric Rehabilitation,* 11, 3, 55-63.

DeFriese, G.H., Konrad, T.R., Woomert, A., Kincade-Norburn, J.E. & Bernard, S. Self-care and quality of life in old age. *Aging and Quality of Life,* (99-117). New York: Springer Publishing Company.

Fiataerone, M.A., O'Neill, E.F., Doyle-Ryan, N., Clements, K.M., Solares, G.R., Nelson, M.E., Roberts, S.B., Kehayias, J.J., Lipsitz, L.A. & Evans, W.J. (1994). Exercise training and nutritional supplementation for physical frailty in very elderly people. *New England Journal of Medicine,* June 23, 1994.

Fonda, S.J., Maddox, G.L., Clipp, E. & Reardon, J. (1996). Design for a longitudinal study of the impact of an enhanced environment on the functioning of frail adults. *The Journal of Applied Gerontology,* 15, 4, 397-413.

Frishkorn, P.H. (1994). Functional assessment as a reimbursement mechanism. *Topics in Geriatric Rehabilitation,* 10, 1, 67-71.

Grant, L.D. (1996). Aspects of ageism on individual and health care providers' responses to healthy aging. *Health and Social Work,* 21, 1, 9-15.

Hellman, E.A., Williams, M.A., Thalken, L. (1996). Modifications of the 7-day activity interview for use among older adults. *The Journal of Applied Gerontology,* 15, 1, 116-131.

Hubley-Kozey, C.L., Wall, J.C. & Hogan, D.B. (1995). Effects of a general exercise program on plantarflexor and dorsiflexor strength and power of older women. *Topics in Geriatric Rehabilitation,* 10, 3, 45-60.

Hughes, M.A., Cooperman, J., Peterson, C. & Duncan, P.W. (1996). Partial weight bearing in the older person. *Topics in Geriatric Rehabilitation,* 11, 3, 1-8.

Lewis, C.B., Lindsay, T. & Scott, C. (1996). Functional assessment in the psychosocial realm. *Topics in Geriatric Rehabilitation,* 11, 4, 64-83.

Mills, K.M., Stewart, A.L., King, A.C., Roitz, K., Sepsis, P.G., Ritter, P.L. & Bortz, W.M. (1996). Factors associated with enrollment of older adults into a physical activity promotion program. *Journal of Aging and Health,* 8, 1, 96-113.

Mills, K.M., Stewart, A.L., Sepsis, P.G. & King, A.C. (1997). Consideration of older adults' preferences for format of physical activity. *Journal of Aging and Physical Activity,* 5, 50-58.

Perkins-Carpenter, B. (1993). *How to Prevent Falls.* New York: St. Martin's Press.

Porter, M.M. & Vandervoort, A.A. (1995). High-intensity strength training for the older adult: A review. *Topics in Geriatric Rehabilitation,* 10, 3, 61-74.

Resnick, B.M. (1991). Geriatric motivation: Clinically helping the elderly to comply. *Journal of Gerontological Nursing,* 17, 5, 17-20.

Ryan, J.W. & Spellbring, A.M. (1996). Implementing strategies to decrease risk of falls in older women. *Journal of Gerontological Nursing,* Dec. 1996, 25-31.

Schaller, K.J. (1996). Tai Chi Chih: An exercise option for older adults. *Journal of Gerontological Nursing,* Oct. 1996, 12-17.

Schilke, J.M. (1991). Slowing the aging process with physical activity. *Journal of Gerontological Nursing,* 17, 6, 4-8.

Seidler, R.D. & Stelmach, G.E. (1995). Reduction in sensorimotor control with age. *Quest,* 47, 386-394.

Shephard, R.J. (1993). Exercise and aging: Extending independence in older adults. *Geriatrics,* 48, 5, 61-64.

Spirduso, W. (1995). *Physical Dimensions of Aging.* Champaign, Ill.: Human Kinetics Publishers.

Spirduso, W. & Asplund, L.A. (1995). Physical activity and cognitive function in the elderly. *Quest,* 47, 395-410.

Strain, L.A. (1996). Lay explanations of chronic illness in later life. *Journal of Aging and Health,* 8, 1, 3-26.

Thornby, M.A. (1995). Balance and falls in the frail older person: A review of the literature. *Topics in Geriatric Rehabilitation,* 11, 2, 35-43.

Tibbitts, M. (1996). Patients who fall: How to predict and prevent injuries. *Geriatrics,* 51, 9, 24-31.

Toomey, T.C. & Seville, J.L. (1994). Assessing functional impairment in elderly patients with chronic pain. *Topics in Geriatric Rehabilitation,* 10, 1, 58-66.

Van Norman, Kay (1995). *Exercise Programming for Older Adults.* Champaign, Ill.: Human Kinetics.

Wagner, E.H., Grothaus, L.C., Hecht, J.A. & LaCroix, A.Z. (1991). Factors associated with participation in a senior health promotion program. *The Gerontologist,* 31, 5, 598-602.

Wolter, L.L., Studenski, S.A. (1996). A clinical synthesis of falls intervention trials. *Topics in Geriatric Rehabilitation,* 11, 3, 9-19.

SUGGESTED READING

American College of Sports Medicine. (1995). *Guidelines for Exercise Testing and Prescription.* Baltimore: Williams & Wilkins.

American Senior Fitness Association. (1995). *Senior Fitness Instructor, Personal Trainer,* and *Long-term Care Training Manuals.* New Smyrna Beach, Fla.

Chodzko-Zajko, W. (Ed.). *Journal of Physical Activity and Aging.* Champaign, Ill.: Human Kinetics.

Clark, J. (1992). *Full Life Fitness.* Champaign, Ill.: Human Kinetics.

Gladwin, L. (1996). Stretching: A valuable component of functional mobility training in activities. *Adaptation & Aging,* 20, 3, 37-47.

Markides, K. (Ed.). *Journal of Aging and Health.* SAGE Periodicals Press.

Sova, R. (1991). *Aquatics: The Complete Reference Guide for Aquatic Fitness Professionals.* Boston: Jones and Bartlett Publishers, Inc.

Spirduso, W. (1995). *Physical Dimensions of Aging.* Champaign, Ill.: Human Kinetics.

Van Norman, K. (1995). *Exercise Programming for Older Adults.* Champaign, Ill.: Human Kinetics.

Welch, G. (1995). Stabilization: An integral part of real life function. *The Senior Fitness Bulletin,* 2, 2.

For further information on home-based exercise brochures and the Permission to M.O.V.E. (Motivation, Opportunity, Verification & Education) campaign, call (406) 994-6316.

glossary

Glossary

adiposity The state of being fat; fatness; obesity.

allergens Substances capable of inducing allergy or specific hypersensitivity.

ataxia Failure of muscular coordination; irregularity of muscular action.

atherosclerosis A common form of arteriosclerosis in which deposits of yellowish plaques (atheromas) containing cholesterol, lipoid material and lipophages are formed within the intima and inner media of arteries.

attending A nonverbal communication skill that gives acknowledgement through posture, eye contact and gestures. It entails being attentive through physical attention and putting the speaker at ease.

atrophy A wasting away; a diminution in the size of a cell, tissue, organ or part.

autoimmune disease Any of a group of disorders in which tissue injury is associated with the body's responses to its own constituents; they may be systemic (e.g., systemic lupus erythematosis) or organ specific (e.g., autoimmune thyroiditis).

autonomic nervous system The portion of the nervous system concerned with regulation of cardiac muscle, smooth muscle and glands; the self-controlling nervous system.

borderline hypertension A term commonly used to describe what the Joint Committee on Detection, Evaluation and Treatment of High Blood Pressure classifies as "high normal;" blood pressure of 130-139 mmHg systolic and 85-89 mmHg diastolic.

cardiac output (CO) The amount of blood pumped by the heart per minute; usually expressed in liters of blood per minute.

catecholamine One of a group of similar compounds having a sympathomimetic action (mimicking the effects of impulses conveyed by the sympathetic nervous system).

carcinogen Any cancer-producing substance.

cirrhosis Liver disease characterized by loss of normal lobular architecture, with fibrosis.

cognitive Pertaining to, or characterized by, that operation of the mind by which we become aware of objects of thought or perception; includes all aspects of perceiving, thinking and remembering.

congestive heart failure A clinical syndrome due to heart disease and characterized by breathlessness, and sodium and water retention, resulting in edema. The congestion can occur in the lungs, in the peripheral circulation or both.

covalent bond Chemical bonds in which electrons can be shared, such as the peptide bonds in proteins.

degenerative changes Changes associated with tissues moving toward a lower or less functionally active form.

demyelinization The destruction or removal of the myelin sheath of a nerve or nerves.

dystrophy Any disorder arising from defective or faulty nutrition, especially the muscular dystrophies.

edema The presence of abnormally large amounts of fluid in the intercellular tissue spaces of the body.

empathic response A response based on the understanding of a person's experience from their perspective; it should acknowledge and increase the awareness of their experience and therefore make them more open to learning.

exercise prescriptions Written directions for the administration of exercise programs.

forced expiratory volume The percentage of vital capacity that can be expired in one second; provides an indication of expiratory power and overall resistance to air movement in the lungs.

gerontologist A specialist in the scientific study of the problems of aging in all their aspects—clinical, biological, historical and sociological.

heart-rate reserve (HRR) The reserve capacity of the heart; the difference between maximal heart rate and resting heart rate. It reflects the heart's ability to increase the rate of beating and cardiac output above resting level to maximal intensity.

homeostasis A tendency toward stability in the normal body states achieved by a system of control mechanisms activated by negative feedback.

hypercholesterolemia An excess of cholesterol in the blood.

hyperlipidemia An excess of lipids in the blood that could be primary, as in disorders of lipid metabolism, or secondary, as in uncontrolled diabetes mellitus.

Karvonen method A method of determining target heart rate that uses heart-rate reserve (maximal heart rate minus resting heart rate).

kyphosis Abnormally increased convexity of the curvature of the thoracic spine (hunchback).

lactic acid A by-product of anaerobic glycolysis known to cause localized, acute muscle fatigue.

liposoluble Able to be dissolved in fats.

maximum voluntary ventilation A dynamic test of ventilatory capacity that requires rapid and deep breathing for 15 seconds (extrapolated to one minute).

maximal oxygen consumption (VO_2max) The point at which oxygen consumption plateaus with an additional workload; represents a person's capacity for the aerobic synthesis of ATP.

neoplastic Pertaining to any new and abnormal growth; specifically when the growth is uncontrolled and progressive.

neurotransmitters A substance that transmits nerve impulses across a synapse (e.g., as acetycholine, norepinephrine).

open kinetic chain (exercises) Exercises in which a muscle or muscle group is isolated to function alone.

orthostatic hypotension A progressive disorder that includes abnormally low blood pressure and symptoms of weakness or fainting upon rising to an erect position; also known as postural hypotension.

peripheral Situated away from the center or central structure.

postural hypotension See *orthostatic hypotension*

residual volume The volume of air that remains in the lungs when an individual exhales as deeply as possible.

rheumatic diseases Any of a variety of disorders marked by inflammation, degeneration or metabolic derangement of the connective tissue structures of the body, especially the joints and related structures (e.g., rheumatoid arthritis, lupus, fibromyalgia).

sciatica A syndrome characterized by pain radiating from the back into the buttock and into the lower extremity along its posterior or lateral aspect, most commonly caused by prolapse of the intervertebral disk. Also refers to pain anywhere along the course of the sciatic nerve.

self-efficacy One's perception of their ability to change or perform specific behaviors.

senescence The process or condition of growing old.

shoulder impingement A shoulder joint injury that arises from the continual use of the arm(s) above the horizontal plane; commonly occurs in the supraspinous muscle at the acromion and coracoacromial ligament.

total peripheral resistance (TPR) The resistance to the passage of blood through the small blood vessels, especially arterioles.

vagus nerve The tenth cranial nerve; parasympathetic, general sensory nerve.

Valsalva maneuver Increase of intrathoracic pressure by forcible exhalation effort against a closed glottis.

vital capacity The total volume of air that can be voluntarily moved in one breath, from full inspiration to maximum expiration, or vice versa.

index

Index

H

Hagberg, J.M., 9, 10

Hayflick, Leonard, 5, 6

Hayflick limit, 6

health belief model, 34

Health-Fitness Gradient

    physically fit-healthy, 14-15

    physically unfit-unhealthy dependent, 16, 17

    physically unfit-unhealthy independent, 15, 17

health history questionnaire, 114

health status, effects of socioeconomic factors on, 31

heart disease

    See cardiovascular disorders

heart-rate assessment, 114-16, 120, 196

    calculating training range, 115-16

    chart for recording, 198

    during fitness walking, 176

    Karvonen (heart-rate reserve) method, 115-16, 135

    and medications, 196

heart-rate reserve (HHR) method (Karvonen), 115-16, 135

heart rhythm disorders, 76

high-density lipoprotein cholesterol, 10

Hochberg, M.C., 86

home-based exercise brochures, 191, 192

Hughes, R.L., 62

Hummert, M.L., 52

humor, in exercise programs, 65-66

Hydralazine, 108

Hydrochlorothiazide (Esidrix, Hydrodiuril, Oretic, Thiuretic), 95

hydrocollator pads, 86

Hydrodiuril, 95

hydrogen-bond cross-links, 6

hydrostatic weighting, 112-13

hypercholesterolemia, 10

hyperlipidemia, 10

hypertension, 10, 77-78

    borderline, 10

    exercise guidelines for, 78

    symptoms, 78

hyperthermia, 96

hyperventilation, 83

hypnotics and tranquilizers, 96

hypoglycemia, 89, 90

hypokalemia, 96

hypotension, orthostatic (postural), 96

I

ibuprofen (Advil, Motrin), 97

Imipramine (Tofranil), 96

immune system functioning, and aging, 6

impairment, 75

Inderal, 95, 108

individualized exercise program, 192

instructor-client relationships, stages of, 56-58

instructor responsibilities, 58-59

instrumental activities of daily living (IADL), 188

insulin-dependent (Type I) diabetes, 89

insulin reaction, 89, 90

intelligence, effects of aging on, 30

intensity, of exercise, 17

    aerobic exercise and, 135-36

    determining, 196

    flexibility training and, 137

    strength training and, 137

intercostal breathing, 150

intermediate activities of daily living (IADL), 106

interval training, 134

    for people with arthritis, 88

    for people with high degree of dyspnea, 83

intrinsic asthma, 79

intrinsic motivation, 44

isolated systolic blood pressure, 78

isometric exercises, 78, 87

Isoproterenol, 80

Isordil, 108

J

Jette, A.M., 75

jogging

    contraindicated for people with arthritis, 88

    as trigger for exercise-induced asthma, 81

joint instability, 86

Joint National Committee of Detection, Evaluation and Treatment of High Blood Pressure, Fifth Report of, 78

Jones, J.C., 119

Jones, M., 117, 121

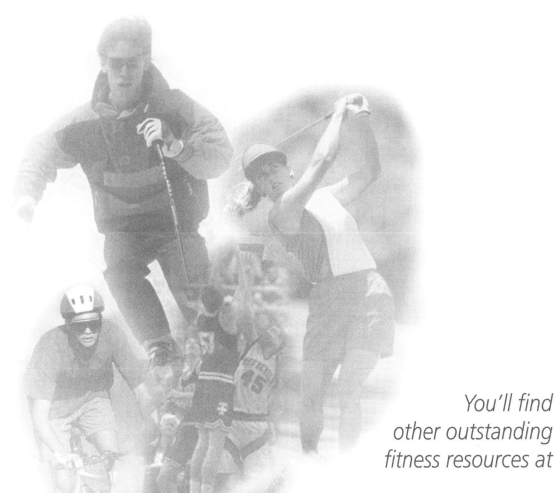